Handbook of On Call Urology.

2nd Edition.

Mr J Clavijo-Eisele (Editor)

Editor and Project manager: Mr. J. Clavijo Eisele, FEBU.

Printer: CreateSpace. North Charleston, SC. USA.

Publisher: Urology Solutions Publishing.

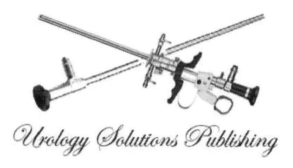

ISBN: 978-0-9931760-3-6

Second Edition: April 2016.

10 9 8 7 6 5 4 3 2

Author Index.

Sr. Sally Larn, RN. Cancer Nurse Specialist in Urology. Diana Princess of Wales Hospital. Grimsby. UK.
Urethral catheter insertion.

Dr. Roberto Molina Escudero. Urologist. Servicio de Urología. Hospital Universitario de Fuenlabrada. Madrid. Spain.
Haematuria. Post-operative complications.

Mr. Werner Mueller. FRCOG. Consultant Gynaecologist. St Hugh's Hospital. Grimsby. UK.
Urinary tract infections during pregnancy.

Mr. Edgar M Paez, FRCS. Consultant Urologist. Freeman Hospital. Newcastle upon Tyne. UK.
Renal and ureteral trauma. Pelvic trauma.

Dr. Ricardo Pou Ferrari. Prof. Agregado de Clínica Ginecológica. Facultad de Medicina. Univ. de la República. Director, Clínica Pou. Montevideo. Uruguay.
Urinary tract infections during pregnancy.

Mr. Peter Rimington, FRCS. Consultant Urological Surgeon. Eastbourne District General Hospital. Eastbourne. UK.
Renal and ureteral trauma.

Mr. Mark Rogers, FRCS. Consultant Urological Surgeon. Scunthorpe General Hospital. Scunthorpe. UK.
Haematuria.

Prof. Abhay Rane, OBE MS FRCS (Urol). Adjunct Professor of Urology at the University of Southern California Los Angeles. US. Consultant Urological Surgeon. Redhill Hospital and Gatwick Park Hospital. Surrey. UK.
Kidney colic.

Mr. Tom Rosenbaum. FRCS. Consultant Urological Surgeon. Ealing Hospital and Clementine Churchill Hospital. London. UK.
Urinary tract infections in children. Acute scrotal pain. Autonomic dysreflexia.

Mr. Samer Salloum, MD, PhD, MRCS. Urology Registrar. Glangwili

General Hospital. Carmarthen. UK.
Infections of the upper urinary tract. Acute cystitis and prostatitis. Male genital infections. Acute urinary retention. Urethral catheter insertion. Suprapubic catheter placement. Haematuria. Paraphimosis. Priapism. Pelvic trauma. External genital trauma. Post-operative complications.

Mr. Guru Balaji Shanmugham, MRCS. Consultant Urologist and Andrologist. Prashanth Hospital and Fortis Hospital. Chennai, India. Paraphimosis.

Mr. Prateek Verma, FRCS. Staff Grade in Urology. Eastbourne District General Hospital. Eastbourne. UK.
Kidney colic. Management of obstructive renal failure. External genital trauma.

Dr. Eduardo Zungri. Consultant Urologist. Clínica Vida and Centro Médico El Castro. Hospital Perpetuo Socorro. Vigo. Spain.
Acute urinary retention. Urethral catheter insertion. Suprapubic catheter placement.

Acknowledgments.

Peter Rimington, Graham Watson and Will Lawrence ushered me into British Urology.

Stuart Tindall has always been supportive, enthusiastic and a balanced critic of my ideas.

Shlomo Raz, Jens Rassweiler, Juan Jubín, Raúl Cepellini Olmos†, Roberto Rocha Brito† and Luis García Guido who were the foundations of my training.

The junior doctors I had the pleasure to work with have provided acute insight into the difficulties of caring for Urology patients with emergency problems.

Several consultant colleagues have written chapters on their area of expertise considerably improving this edition.

Mr. Jorge Clavijo-Eisele

Table of Contents.

Introduction.

This book is a collection of solutions for Acute Urology problems.

It will hopefully make your life easier and will help you to learn the tasks required to provide good emergency care in the speciality.

All superfluous information or controversies have been deliberately omitted.

Many acute patients have co-morbidities so you will have to use the information provided as part of the overall care.

Neither this book nor any other will provide you with good judgement or experience. You will hopefully develop both and I expect the book to be of support and a guide.

Most of the principles of Good Medical Practice apply to acute Urology. Be safe and provide the solution that best suits the patient's interest.

If you are safely spared one call into Hospital because someone has read this book, it will have fulfilled its purpose.

Good luck and enjoy the book!

Mr Jorge Clavijo
New Waltham
Summer 2016

To Andy and Martin
My arrows into the future.
And to Rossana
The bow.

Handbook of On Call Urology.

In theory there is no difference between theory and practice;
in practice there is.

CHAPTER 1. Infections of the Urinary Tract.

Definition.
A urinary tract infection (UTI) is the invasion and reaction of the urinary tract to the disease producing organisms and their toxins. The reaction usually includes inflammation of the involved organ. In men these infections usually also involve the genital organs.

The majority of these cases will be dealt with in the community with just symptom management in the least severe scenario and short courses of antibiotics for the rest. Most UTIs can progress to urinary sepsis. This is a serious condition with high morbidity and mortality.

UTIs are also the most frequent healthcare associated ("iatrogenic") infections.

Classification of urinary tract infections:
1. Uncomplicated lower UTI (cystitis).
2. Uncomplicated pyelonephritis.
3. Complicated UTI with or without urosepsis including: pyelonephritis, pyonephrosis, abscesses, prostatitis, epididymitis and orchitis. UTIs on a structural or functional abnormal organ or with an underlying disease that compromises the patient's immune response.
4. Urethritis and STDs.

1.1. Infections of the upper urinary tract.

Mr S Salloum and Mr J Clavijo.

Definition.

Pyelonephritis: infection of the renal pelvis and kidney without obstruction.

Pyonephrosis: infection of the renal pelvis and kidney in an obstructed system. This leads to the collection of white blood cells, bacteria, and debris (pus and pyuria) in the system above the obstruction. Basically an infected hydronephrosis. The kidney function is compromised. It is an advanced stage of obstructive pyelonephritis.

Other presentations may include abscesses in or adjacent to the kidney. The presence of gas ("emphysematous") produced by infective agents can be seen in scans. The inflammatory or fibrotic reaction to the infections is called "xanthogranulomatous" (and is rare). The first two account for the majority of cases.

Aetiology.

The mechanism involves either an ascending urinary infection or the haematogenous spread of bacteria. As many of these presentations will be complicated urinary tract infections, the underlying cause will also need to be investigated and treated.

The most frequent organisms are Enterobacteria, mainly E Coli, Pseudomonas and gram positive cocci (Staphylococcus and Enterococcus).

Diagnosis.

1. History: it should look at identifying the possible source of infection, asking for symptoms such as pain and dysuria. Frequency and urgency may also occur. In patients catheterised or in elderly patients the only feature may be decreased consciousness or confusion. Other symptoms: fever, flank pain, nausea, vomiting, haematuria, frequency, urgency, systemic symptoms (asthenia, anorexia, fatigue).

Differential: rule out causes of acute abdomen. In patients at the extremes of age, the presentation may be atypical.

The classic presentation in acute pyelonephritis is:
- Fever.
- Costovertebral angle pain.
- Pyuria.

Past medical history: stones, previous UTI or a catheter. Congenital malformations. Surgery. Diabetes and immune disorders. Drug history: immune suppressants.

2. Physical examination: fever, hypotension, pallor, palpable kidneys that can be painful.

3. Investigations:
Blood: samples should be taken for culture of blood (if pyrexia >38° C) and also blood sent for renal function and electrolytes (U&E) and a full blood count (FBC). Inflammatory markers: CRP, ESR, procalcitonin.

Imaging: the objective is to identify patients with obstructed kidneys whose pyonephrosis requires drainage. The radiological investigation of choice will depend upon local resources, but will be either ultrasound scanning (Fig. 1.1) or CT (Fig. 1.2 and 1.3). There are advantages with both investigations. Ultrasound can identify a hydronephrotic kidney with no exposure to radiation. It can also be freely used with no contraindications, ideally in the emergency area and by the Urology team. CT scanning on the other hand involves radiation exposure (contraindicated in early pregnancy), but can also, with greater reliability identify calculi, the most common cause of ureteric obstruction. On CT look for areas of perfusion defects in pyelonephritis. As mentioned above, also look for abscesses, gas, and fibrosis and assess the contralateral kidney.

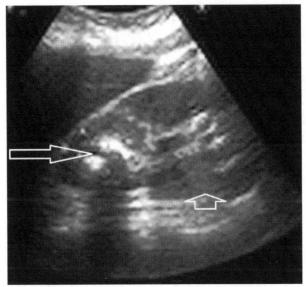

Fig. 1.1. Ultrasound scan showing pelvi-calyceal dilatation (short arrow) and upper pole stones with posterior shadow (long arrow).

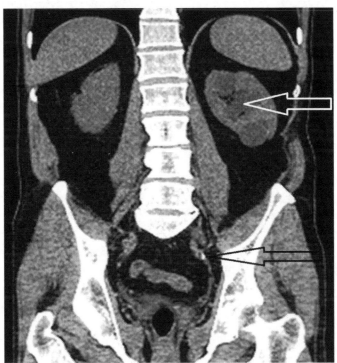

Fig. 1.2. Coronal view of CT with left ureteric stone (black arrow) and left pelvi-calyceal dilatation (white arrow).

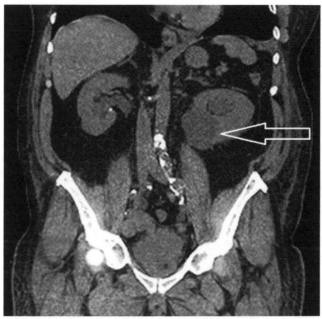

Fig. 1.3. CT with left renal abscess (white arrow).

Others: urine dip and culture with sensitivity.

Treatment.
Medical: in the collapsed patient with urosepsis intra-venous (i/v) access and fluid resuscitation are required urgently. Further management will be better done in ITU. Follow local resuscitation protocol.

Provide analgesia and anti-pyretics. Before cultures are available, consider a beta lactam (Amoxicillin) associated with aminoglycoside (Gentamycin) i/v, or a quinolone (Ciprofloxacin) either i/v or oral according to patient status. Regimes: Ciprofloxacin 500mg BID for 2 weeks or Cefotaxime 1-2g TDS or Ceftriaxone 500mg QDS 14 days or Gentamycin 3-5 mg/kg OD. If there is no clinical response: Tazocin 4.5 g TDS.

Antibiotic treatment depends upon local guidance as local prescribing patterns do affect sensitivity. The length of treatment will depend on the severity of the infection. It will be between 7 and 14 days for simple pyelonephritis, up to 21 days in pyonephrosis, or even continuing until the predisposing cause has been eradicated.

Patients without dilatation (by CT or USS) and without systemic compromise may be considered for a trial of closely supervised outpatient treatment.

Special scenarios:
a. Indwelling catheters or nephrostomy:
- Don't treat asymptomatic bacteriuria.
- If pyrexial or foul urine, get culture and sensitivity and treat accordingly.
- The course of antibiotics should last 7-14 days.

b. Spinal cord injury:
- Full urodynamic assessment should be done with aseptic urine or the lowest achievable bacterial load (and under antibiotic coverage). Non urgent.
- Ensure the bladder is empty with no residual volume.
- Don't treat asymptomatic bacteriuria.

Surgical: after immediate management with analgesia and antibiotics the subsequent step is to identify the predisposing cause and identify which patients will need immediate or delayed interventions. The single main cause of morbidity and mortality in UTIs is procrastination so act swiftly and effectively.

In the case of patients with urinary tract infections that are having any form of intervention, suitable antibiotic treatment must be commenced before the procedure, so the likely passage of bacteria into the circulation and the effects from this are minimised. For patients with urinary retention and sepsis the passage of a urethral catheter will allow drainage and aid resolution of the infection.
The treatment in an emergency setting will also depend on services available locally.

A **nephrostomy**[1] will allow drainage of pyonephrosis, but other options are possible depending on the clinical scenario. A retrograde ureteral catheter (open end) or **JJ stenting**[2] may be sufficient to drain an obstructed system. With the latter approach bacteraemia

---

[1] See Renal colic chapter (2.4).
[2] See Renal colic chapter (2.4).

may be more frequent than with antegrade interventions. Drain collections either surgically or percutaneous (image guided). Do not waste time.

In exceptional cases, the decision may be to attempt treatment of a calculus with ureteroscopy and lithotripsy. If the patient does not improve in spite of drainage, an emergency nephrectomy may become necessary, with considerable morbidity and mortality in septic patients.

Once the infection has subsided plan elective de-obstruction of hydronephrotic units.

Urinary stones: among patients with staghorn calculi 80% have UTIs, so plan complete removal of the stone and treatment of the infection. If the stone can't be removed, then start long term antibiotic therapy (Ciprofloxacin 500mg BID for a month).

Complications.
Sepsis, shock and multi-organ failure if the infection is not controlled, with a mortality rate circa 80%.

Outcomes.
Complicated UTIs respond to the basic principles of infection treatment: drain and provide adequate antibiotics. Maintain hydration levels to optimal standards and correct intervening co-morbidities effectively and promptly.

Additional reading:
1. Urinary tract infections in adults. National Institute for health and Care Excellence (NICE). https://www.nice.org.uk/guidance/qs90. On 20/03/2016.
2. Adult UTIs. American Urological Association. https://www.auanet.org/common/pdf/education/Adult-UTI.pdf. On 20/03/2016.
3. Initial treatment of pyonephrosis using percutaneous nephrostomy. Value of the technique. Lledó García E, Herranz Amo F, Moncada Iribarren I, Verdu Tartajo F, Duran Merino R, de Palacio España A, González Chamorro F, Camuñez Alonso F, Echenagusia Belda A, Simo Muerza G, et al. Arch Esp Urol. 1993 Oct; 46(8):711-8.
4. Urological Infections. European Association of Urology Guidelines. http://uroweb.org/wp-content/uploads/EAU-Guidelines-Urological-Infections-v2.pdf. On 20/03/2016.
5. Imaging of urinary tract infection in the adult. Browne RF, Zwirewich C, Torreggiani WC. Eur Radiol. 2004 Mar; 14 Suppl 3:E168-83.

1.2. Acute cystitis and prostatitis.

Lower urinary tract infections.

Mr S Salloum and Mr J Clavijo.

A. Acute bacterial cystitis.

Definition.
Superficial infection which affects the epithelial lining of the bladder. This infection is frequent in women, without malformations of the urinary system, functional anomalies or risk factors (Simple Acute Cystitis). Approximately 50% of adult women will have at least one episode of cystitis, an in half of these women there will be at least one recurrence. This incidence increases in young women, at the beginning of their sexual life, with changes in the vaginal flora, an increased vaginal pH and with the use of spermicides. Postmenopausal hormonal changes increase the risk of UTIs in 60% of women and this is related to a loss of vaginal and urethral trophism.

Aetiology.
30 times more frequent in women than in men. Most cystitis is caused by a single etiologic agent. Gram negative bacteria are responsible for most cases, and the most common is the Escherichia Coli, 80% of cases. Other responsible uropathogens are: Proteus mirabilis, Klebsiella pneumoniae, Enterococcus faecalis and Staphylococcus saprophyticus. Candida in immunocompromised patients, long term antibiotic therapy, DM patients or on steroids.
The presence of intracellular bacterial communities of Escherichia Coli in the bladder urothelium can be the cause of recurrent urinary infections in the paediatric population.

Diagnosis.
1. History: dysuria, frequency, urgency, suprapubic pain, haematuria. Gynaecology history: discharge or vaginal irritation.
Past medical history: UTIs, relation with intercourse, constipation.
Drug history: hormones and immune-suppressants.

2. Physical examination: rule out acute abdomen. Vaginal trophism. Inspect urethra for diverticula. Prolapse.

3. Investigations:
Imaging: USS with PVR for recurrent cystitis (not urgent).

Others: diagnosis is made by symptoms and urine dip analysis. If leucocytes and nitrates are found, empiric antibiotics must be started. MSU and C&S are indicated in complex or recurrent cases. Flexible cystoscopy for recurrent UTIs (not urgent).

Treatment.
Medical.
25 to 40% of female cystitis resolve without medication. Antibiotics should be chosen according to prevalent local flora and sensibility profile. Nitrofurantoin and Fosfomycin are usually considered first line, due to the high sensitivity (over 90% of Escherichia Coli strains). They should be effective for the vast majority of cases:
Nitrofurantoin 100 mg BID for 3 days.
Fosfomycin 3 g (women only) single dose (SD).

In case of Candida infection: Fluconazole 200–400 mg orally, OD for 2 weeks. And always refer for further studies.

Complications.
Cystitis can escalate to pyelonephritis and sepsis, especially in immune-compromised patients. Haematuria, AUR, dyspareunia.

Outcomes.
Generally good with early recognition and treatment. In recurrent cases, treat the present episode and always refer for elective evaluation and treatment.

B. Acute bacterial prostatitis.

Definition.
Bacterial acute inflammation of the prostate tissue. It affects men of all ages, mainly between 35 and 50 years old. Prostatitis is the most frequent prostate disorder among men below 50.

Aetiology.

Cystitis and cysto-prostatitis in the male are **always** suspicious of an underlying anatomical or functional disorder, so treat and organise further studies. Normally due to Enterobacteria (65 to 80% of all cases), but gram positive cocci, anaerobics and MRSA can also be involved. Other microorganisms such as Chlamydia, Mycoplasma and Trichomonas can also be found particularly in afebrile patients. Bacterial Prostatic Colonization (BPC) is a frequent finding in obstructed and catheterised patients.

Diagnosis.

1. History: chills, fever, nausea, vomiting, perineal and suprapubic pain, frequency, urgency, intermittent stream and urinary retention, hypogastric pain or mass (AUR), urethral secretion, enlarged painful testes.

Past medical history: predisposed by a previous UTI, phimosis, unprotected anal intercourse or a catheter. Infravesical obstruction. TRUS Prostate biopsy. Urological or ano-rectal procedures. Drug history: immune-suppressants.

2. Physical examination: urinary retention, hypogastric pain or mass, urethral secretion, enlarged painful testes or epididymii, peno-scrotal skin inflammation. On rectal examination (Fig. 1.4): tender, enlarged, soft prostate that may be irregular and warm. You may want to defer DRE to avoid exacerbation of symptoms and bacteraemia.

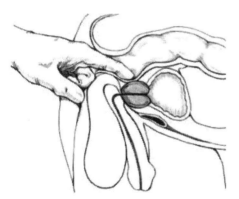

Fig. 1.4. The diagnosis is clinical (rectal examination) and by urine test.

3. Investigations:

Blood: FBC, blood culture if pyrexial. Don't do a PSA, prostatitis cause high PSAs so treat the infection and check PSA 4 weeks after the infection has resolved.

Imaging: USS with post void residual urine measurement.

Others: dipstick: look for leukocytes and nitrates. MSU and C&S (culture and sensitivity): presence of bacteria and sensitivity.

Treatment.
Medical.
Ciprofloxacin 500 mg BID for 2-4 weeks. For the patients who are septic: IV Amoxicillin 500 mg-1g TDS + Gentamycin 3-5 mg/kg OD till the systemic infection resolves, then Ciprofloxacin 500 mg BID orally to complete 4 weeks. Add alpha blockers if voiding symptoms are present or suspected.

Surgical.
Treat urinary retention: short term urinary catheter or preferably a suprapubic catheter.

Complications.
Prostatic abscess (Fig. 1.5 and 1.6) or failure of treatment (confirm by CT scan).

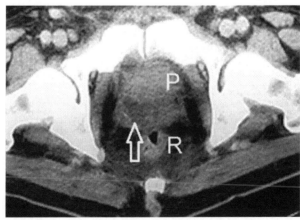

Fig. 1.5. CT showing prostatic abscess (arrow). P: prostate. R: rectum.

Treatment is trans-rectal drainage, transurethral incision or trans-rectal aspiration.

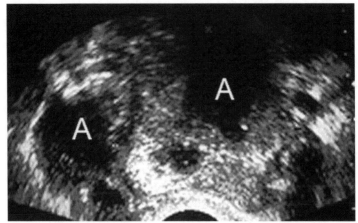

Fig. 1.6. Trans-rectal USS showing prostatic abscesses (A).

Outcomes.

Generally good. Must be electively assessed for lower urinary tract conditions.

Additional reading:

1. Urological Infections. European Association of Urology Guidelines. http://uroweb.org/wp-content/uploads/EAU-Guidelines-Urological-Infections-v2.pdf. On 20/03/2016.
2. Diagnosis and treatment of acute uncomplicated cystitis. Colgan R, Williams M. Am Fam Physician. 2011 Oct 1; 84(7):771-6.
3. Prostatitis: diagnosis and treatment. Sharp VJ, Takacs EB, Powell CR. Am Fam Physician. 2010 Aug 15; 82(4):397-406.
4. Diagnosis, treatment and follow-up of community-acquired bacterial infections of the urinary system of men and women (acute cystitis and acute pyelonephritis) and of the genital system of men (acute prostatitis): general remarks. Bruyère F, Cariou G, Boiteux JP, Hoznek A, Mignard JP, Escaravage L, Bernard L, Sotto A, Soussy CJ, Coloby P; le CIAFU. Prog Urol. 2008 Mar; 18 Suppl 1:4-8.
5. Antibiotics versus placebo in the treatment of women with uncomplicated cystitis: a metaanalysis of randomized controlled trials. Falagas ME, Kotsantis IK, Vouloumanou EK, et al. J Infect. 2009; 58(2): 91-102.
6. Community-acquired methicillin resistant Staphylococcus aureus: a new aetiological agent of prostatic abscess. Abreu D, Arroyo C, Suarez R, Campolo H, Izaguirre J, Decia R, Machado M, Carvalhal GF, Clavijo J. BMJ Case Rep. 2011 May 12. PMID: 22696740.
7. Urinary tract infections in adults. National Institute for health and Care Excellence (NICE). https://www.nice.org.uk/guidance/qs90. On 20/03/2016.
8. Adult UTIs. American Urological Association. https://www.auanet.org/common/pdf/education/Adult-UTI.pdf. On 20/03/2016.
9. International Clinical Practice Guidelines for the Treatment of Acute Uncomplicated Cystitis and Pyelonephritis in Women. Infectious Diseases Society of America; European Society for Microbiology and Infectious Diseases. Clin Infect Dis. 2011 Mar 1; 52(5): e103-20.

1.3. Male genital infections.

Mr S Salloum and Mr J Clavijo.

The different male genital organs (Fig. 1.7) can undergo infections that vary in presentation and management. Hence each condition will be described separately.

A. Epididymitis with or without orchitis.

Definition.
It is an inflammatory condition of the epididymis sometimes involving the testis. Usually secondary to a UTI caused by bacteria. This is a serious acute urological emergency.

Aetiology.
Generally Gram negative rods (enterobacteria). It can also be produced by STD organisms like Neisseria, Mycoplasma and Chlamydia. More rarely mumps or TB orchitis. The infection starts in the urine (UTI) or urethra (STI) and advances retrograde in the genital tract to the epididymis first and testicle last. Rarely haematogenous.

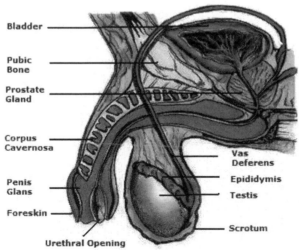

Fig. 1.7. Diagram of the male genital tract.

Like any other infection, it can progress rapidly in immunocompromised patients (frail, elderly, diabetics, alcohol and drug abusers, on steroids, HIV, chemo, etc.).

Diagnosis.
1. History: fever, rigors, scrotal swelling, scrotal pain radiating to the groin, lower abdominal pain, erythema of the skin. Systemically look for mumps, TB, congenital malformations, STDs, urinary infection, recent instrumentation.

2. Physical examination: painful, heavy testis with inflammation. Pain can be relieved by elevation (Prehn's sign). Cremasteric reflex present (stroke the medial aspect of the thigh and see a contraction of the cremaster muscle that elevates the testis). Check for prostatitis in rectal examination. Rule out mumps parotiditis. Examine all the perineum for Fournier's.

Differential: be aware of testicular torsion where the pain is more acute (sudden) and localised in the testis. If not sure, testicular exploration is the safest option.

3. Investigations:
Blood: FBC, culture if pyrexial.

Imaging: scrotal USS, which shows enlarged and vascular epididymis. Look for abscess.

Other: dip stick, MSU. STD screen in young patients or if there is suspicion of an infective contact (not urgent).

Treatment.
Medical.
Antibiotic therapy: Ciprofloxacin 500mg BID for 14 days. Alternatively Doxycycline 100mg OD for 14 days (if an STD is suspected). As always adjust antibiotic treatment when culture results become available (MSU, blood, STDs).

If the patient is systemically unwell: i/v Ceftriaxone 500mg-1g QDS +/- Gentamycin 3-5 mg/kg till the systemic infection resolves, then oral Ciprofloxacin 500 BID to complete 14 days. Supportive therapy includes bed rest, anti-inflammatories, scrotal elevation, and ice packs.

Surgical: if the USS shows an abscess, drain it promptly.

Complications.
Chronic epididymitis: the epididymis is thickened and may be tender. Treatment: antibiotics or epididymectomy in severe cases.

Obstructive infertility. Hydrocele. Abscess formation.

Orchitis: swollen, tender testis. Cause: extension of the epididymal infection, mumps, tuberculosis, syphilis, autoimmune process. Mumps orchitis usually happens in 3rd-4th day of parotiditis and can result in testicular atrophy (60%) and infertility. Treatment: supportive therapy as above.

Outcomes.
Good with treatment.

B. Balanitis.

Definition.
Inflammation of the glans penis. Balano-posthitis includes also inflammation of the foreskin (Fig. 1.8).

Aetiology.
Trauma, bacterial infection, candidiasis.   More prevalent in uncircumcised men with inadequate personal hygiene. Diabetes, obesity.

Diagnosis.
1. History: pain, itching, erythema and swelling of the glans penis, discharge, voiding difficulties.   Balano-posthitis is a cause of phimosis and paraphimosis which might need surgical treatment (usually with circumcision). Past medical history: phimosis.

2. Physical examination: extent of lesions. Presence of inguinal lymph nodes. Ulcers suspicious of STDs.

3. Investigations:
Culture the discharge, including bacterial, mycotic and viral agents.

STD screen in young patients or if there is suspicion (not urgent). In adults check diabetes (HbA1c).

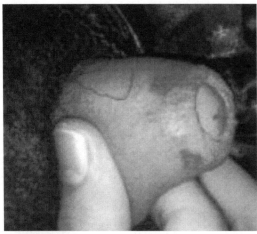

Fig. 1.8. Clinical findings in balano-posthitis. Ask patient to retract the foreskin to avoid pain.

Treatment.
Medical.
- Treat with antibiotics. Start with Trimethoprim.
- Betamethasone 1% cream, for 30 days to relieve the symptoms. Rest, ice, compression, elevation, NSAIDs (RICEN) as well.
- Circumcision for recurrent balano-posthitis or if there is phimosis (not urgent).
- Biopsy if suspicion of carcinoma in situ (Bowen, Queyrat) also elective.

Complications.
Phimosis.

Outcomes.
Good with treatment. As it will be recurrent, organize treatment of any predisposing factor.

C. **Urethritis.**

Definition.
Usually purulent urethral discharge associated with a STD. Dysuria and inflammation of the urethra (Fig. 1.9).

Aetiology & classification.

- Nongonococcal Urethritis (NGU) agents: Chlamydia trachomatis, Ureaplasma, Mycoplasma. Rarely Trichomonas.
- Gonorrhoea: Neisseria gonorrhoea.

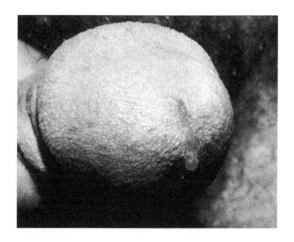

Fig. 1.9. Urethral discharge.

Diagnosis.
1. History: frequency, urgency, burning sensation with voiding, mucous discharge. With gonorrhoea: profuse and purulent discharge. But 25% can be asymptomatic.

Past medical history: STDs, contacts.

2. Physical examination: urethral discharge. Check for epididymitis/orchitis and inguinal lymph nodes. Temperature.

3. Investigations:
Blood: STD screen according to local guidance (not urgent) including HIV, hepatitis B+C and syphilis.

Others: send for culture and analysis: urethral swab and urine.
- Urine dip: positive dipstick for leucocyte esterase on first passed urine (FPU).
- Microscopy of either a urethral swab or first-void urine sample. (Gram stained urethral smear).
- Urine for nucleic acid amplification tests (NAATs) for Chlamydia trachomatis and N. gonorrhoea.

Treatment.
Gonorrhoea: Ceftriaxone 250 mg by intramuscular injection (single

dose) or oral Cefixime 400 mg stat.

Non gonococcal urethritis: Azithromycin 1g orally stat or doxycycline 100 mg BID orally for 7 days.

Patient and contacts standard STD advice.

Complications.
Reiter's syndrome (joint pain, conjunctivitis), recurring urethritis sometimes non-infectious, epididymo-orchitis, urethral stricture.

Outcomes.
Good with treatment.

D. Fournier's gangrene.

Definition.
It is a necrotizing cellulitis and fasciitis of the external genitalia and perineum.

Aetiology.
A combination of micro-organisms (particularly anaerobic) causes an infection that spreads quickly and causes necrosis of skin, subcutaneous tissue, and muscle.

Incidence and prevalence: men are ten times more likely than women to develop Fournier's gangrene. Women who have had a pus-producing bacterial infection (abscess) in the vaginal area, episiotomy, septic abortion, or hysterectomy are susceptible. Rarely, children may develop Fournier's gangrene as a complication from a burn, circumcision, or an insect bite.

Risk factors: men with alcoholism, diabetes mellitus, leukaemia, morbid obesity, immune system disorders and intravenous drug users are at increased risk for developing Fournier's gangrene. The condition also can develop as a complication of surgery.

Fournier's gangrene develops when bacteria infect the body through a wound, usually in the perineum (anal, rectal or urogenital areas). Existing immune system deficiencies help the infection to spread quickly, producing a disease that destroys the skin and superficial and deep fascia of the genital area. The corpora cavernosa, testicles, and urethra are not usually affected.

Classification.
- Anterior: involves external genitals and anterior abdominal wall (Fig. 1.10). Usually of urological origin.
- Posterior: involves the posterior perineum behind the scrotum and the peri-rectal area (Fig. 1.11). Usually of anal or rectal origin.

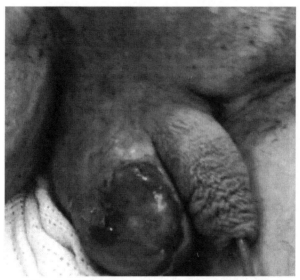

Fig. 1.10. Anterior Fournier's gangrene.

Diagnosis.
1. History: early physical symptoms of Fournier's gangrene may not indicate the severity of the condition. Pain sometimes diminishes as the disease progresses. It is a clinical diagnosis. It is a urological emergency that needs experienced senior management.
   Past medical history: immune suppression.

2. Physical examination: check extent of fasciitis and mark with permanent marker. Look for necrotic areas and areas of crepitation (gas). Investigate initial focus. Devitalised and discoloured (grey-black) tissue; pus weeping from entry site. Fever and drowsiness (lethargy). Increasing genital pain and

redness (erythema). Severe genital pain accompanied by tenderness and swelling of the penis and scrotum. Characteristic foul odour.

3. Investigations:
Blood: FBC, U&E, CRP, ABG.

Imaging: CT to assess all abdominal and pelvic organs and abdominal wall.

Others: urine and exudates cultures. Blood culture, particularly if pyrexial.

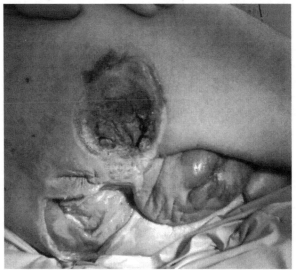

Fig. 1.11. Posterior Fournier's gangrene.

Treatment.
Medical.
In collapsed patients, apply resuscitation protocol. Antibiotics (often double or triple drug therapy) along with aggressive surgical removal of the diseased tissue are required immediately for an optimal outcome. Amoxicillin + Gentamycin + Metronidazole at full doses is the usual regime, which should be tailored when the results of pus and blood cultures are available.

Surgical.
Immediate wide debridement resecting all compromised and

suspicious tissue. Abundant saline and antiseptic wash.

Hyperbaric oxygen therapy (HBO) can be used as an adjuvant, as can topical hygroscopic substances if the patient recovers.

Complications.
Incomplete debridement (surgical removal of dead tissue) allows wound infection to continue to spread. In this event, follow-up surgery is performed. Without early treatment, bacterial infection enters the bloodstream and will cause sepsis, respiratory failure, and death. Fournier's gangrene is usually fatal if the infection becomes systemic.

Outcomes.
Mortality rates are high (20%) and escalate with worse performance status. In those who survive, reconstructive procedures may be needed later.

Additional reading:
1. British Association for Sexual Health and HIV Guidelines. http://www.bashh.org/BASHH/Guidelines/Guidelines/BASHH/Guidelines/Guidelines.aspx?hkey=072c83ed-0e9b-44b2-a989-7c84e4fbd9de. On 20/03/2016.
2. Hyperbaric oxygen treatment in urology. Gallego Vilar D, García Fadrique G, Povo Martín IJ, Miralles Aguado J, Garau Perelló C, Sanchis Verdú L, Gimeno Argente V, Bosquet Sanz M, Aliaga MR, Claramonte Ramón FJ, Gallego Gómez J. Arch Esp Urol. 2011 Jul; 64(6):507-16.
3. Urological Infections. European Association of Urology Guidelines. http://uroweb.org/wp-content/uploads/EAU-Guidelines-Urological-Infections-v2.pdf. On 20/03/2016.
4. Fournier's gangrene and its emergency management. Thwaini A, Khan A, Malik A, Cherian J, Barua J, Shergill I, Mammen K. Postgrad Med J. 2006 Aug; 82(970):516-9.
5. Sexually Transmitted Diseases. Centers for Disease Control and Prevention. http://www.cdc.gov/std/. On 20/03/2016.
6. Adult UTIs. American Urological Association. https://www.auanet.org/common/pdf/education/Adult-UTI.pdf. On 20/03/2016.
7. Urinary tract infections in adults. National Institute for health and Care Excellence (NICE). https://www.nice.org.uk/guidance/qs90. On 20/03/2016.

1.4. Urinary tract infections during pregnancy.

Mr W Muller and Dr R Pou-Ferrari.

Definition.
Significant bacteriuria is two consecutive voided urine specimens that grow $> 10^5$ cfu/mL of the same bacterial species on quantitative culture; or a single catheterised specimen that grows $> 10^5$ cfu/mL of an uropathogen.

In a pregnant woman with symptoms compatible with UTI, bacteriuria is considered significant if a voided or catheterised urine specimen grows $> 10^3$ cfu/mL of an uropathogen.

All pregnant women need to be screened in the first trimester and treated if significant bacteriuria is found.

Aetiology.
The occurrence of urinary tract infections during pregnancy is common and may be predisposed by the physiological and anatomical changes that occur during pregnancy. The physiological changes include hormonal factors, progesterone has an inhibitory action on smooth muscle in general, including the ureter. This is why UTI predisposition begins early in gestation. Hydroureteronephrosis during pregnancy starts around the seventh week and resolves by 8 weeks after delivery. The right system is the more affected.

Symptomatic infection occurs in about 1-4% of pregnant women. 20-40% of women with asymptomatic significant bacteriuria have pyelonephritis during pregnancy (mostly in the 3rd trimester) leading to premature labour.

Classification.
- Asymptomatic bacteriuria.
- Cystitis.
- Pyelonephritis.

Diagnosis.
1. History: the clinical presentation of UTIs is similar in pregnant and non-pregnant patients. Fever, loin pain and pyuria for pyelonephritis. Dysuria and frequency for cystitis.

Past medical history: recurrent UTIs, urological malformations, urinary operations or diseases (lithiasis, Fig. 1.12). Drug and medication history for immune suppression.

2.   Physical examination yields little due to the pregnancy.

3.   Investigations:
Blood: FBC, U&Es.

Imaging: USS to assess dilatation (Fig. 1.13), renal stones, post void residual. Ionising radiation should be avoided, especially in 1st and 2nd trimesters if at all possible.

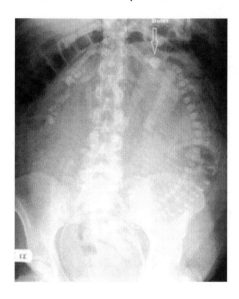

Fig. 1.12. KUB x-ray of a pregnant woman (3rd trimester) with left pyelonephritis secondary to a renal stone (white arrow).

Others: urine dip and MSU. Although we would send off a specimen in any case, start treatment based on symptoms and a dipstick positive for leukocytes and nitrates.

Treatment.
Medical.
Cephalosporins and pencillins will be the first line choices as tetracyclines, quinolones and sulphonamides are contraindicated.

Asymptomatic bacteriuria is treated with a 7-day course based on sensitivity testing. For recurrent infections (symptomatic or asymptomatic), Cephalexin, 125-250 mg/day, or Nitrofurantoin (2nd and 3rd trimesters only), 50 mg/day, may be used for prophylaxis, as well as cranberry juice and probiotic preparations.

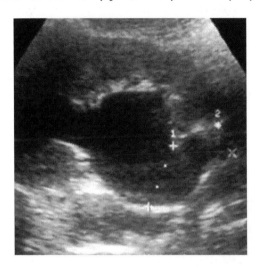

Fig. 1.13. USS image of hydro-ureteronephrosis during pregnancy. 1: dilated pelvis. 2.: dilated proximal ureter.

Antibiotic regimes for significant bacteriuria:
- Co-amoxiclav 625mg TDS 3-5 days.
- Cephalexin 500 mg TDS 3-5 days.
- Fosfomycin 3g single dose (avoid trimethoprim in 1st trimester and sulfamethoxazole in 3rd trimester).

Treatment of pyelonephritis in pregnancy:
- Ceftriaxone 1-2 g IV or IM OD.
- Aztreonam 1 g IV BID.
- Piperacillin-Tazobactam 3.375-4.5 g IV QDS.
- Imipenem-Cilastatin 500 mg IV QDS.
- Ampicillin 2 g IV QDS + Gentamicin 3-5 mg/kg/day IV.

Treatment should last 7-10 days. Can be as outpatient if there is no nausea and vomiting but in severe cases admit and start IV treatment till the symptoms are relieved and then change to oral treatment to complete 2 weeks.

Most antibiotics carry a very small risk of teratogenesis. UTIs during pregnancy can lead to serious consequences if left untreated. The antibiotics commonly used have not been found to be associated with a significantly increased risk of birth defects when used during pregnancy.

Surgical.

For cases of ureter obstruction, stenting or rarely nephrostomy should be considered.

Complications.

Mainly pre-term labour, but any other complication possible in a non-pregnant patient can also happen during pregnancy.

Outcomes.

Very good when treated early and in the absence of co-morbidities.

Additional reading:

1. Urological Infections. European Association of Urology Guidelines. http://uroweb.org/wp-content/uploads/EAU-Guidelines-Urological-Infections-v2.pdf. On 20/03/2016.
2. Management of suspected bacterial UTI in adults. Scottish Intercollegiate Guidelines Network. http://www.sign.ac.uk/guidelines/fulltext/88/recommendations.html. On 20/03/2016.
3. Treatments for symptomatic urinary tract infections during pregnancy. Vazquez JC, Abalos E. Cochrane Database Syst Rev. 2011. Jan 19; (1).
4. Safety and efficacy of cranberry (vaccinium macrocarpon) during pregnancy and lactation. Dugoua JJ, Seely D, Perri D, Mills E, Koren G. Can J Clin Pharmacol. 2008 Winter; 15(1).
5. Urinary tract infections in pregnancy. Lee M, Bozzo P, Einarson A, Koren G. Can Fam Physician. 2008 Jun; 54(6):853-4.
6. Different antibiotic regimens for treating asymptomatic bacteriuria in pregnancy. Guinto VT, De Guia B, Festin MR, Dowswell T. Cochrane Database Syst Rev. 2010 Sep 8; (9).
7. Recurrent urinary tract infection. Epp A, Larochelle A, Lovatsis D, Walter JE, Easton W, Farrell SA, Girouard L, Gupta C, Harvey MA, Robert M, Ross S, Schachter J, Schulz JA, Wilkie D, Ehman W, Domb S, Gagnon A, Hughes O, Konkin J, Lynch J, Marshall C, Society of Obstetricians and Gynaecologists of Canada. J Obstet Gynaecol Can. 2010 Nov; 32(11): 1082-101.

1.5. Urinary tract infections in children.

Mr T Rosenbaum and Mr J Clavijo.

Definition.
A UTI is the invasion and reaction of the urinary tract to the disease producing organisms and their toxins. The reaction usually includes inflammation of the involved organ.

Aetiology.
Usually gram negative rods (Enterobacteria) when linked to a congenital urological problem. Gram positive cocci in blood borne cases.

Paediatric UTI is the most common cause of fever of unknown origin in boys aged < 3 years.

Classification.
- Severe UTI: fever of > 39°C, feeling of being ill, persistent vomiting, and moderate or severe dehydration.

- Simple UTI: mild pyrexia, but the child is able to take fluids and oral medication. The child is only slightly or not dehydrated and has a good level of compliance. When a low level of compliance is expected, all cases should be managed as a severe UTI.

Diagnosis.
1. History: the clinical presentation of UTIs in infants and young children can vary from fever to gastrointestinal complaints (vomiting and diarrhoea) and lower or upper urinary tract symptoms. When they are older than 2 years, frequent voiding, dysuria and suprapubic, abdominal or lumbar pain may appear with or without fever. Presentation can include failure to thrive, hypothermia, irritability, jaundice, poor feeding, sepsis, enuresis, gross haematuria, meningismus, strong-smelling urine, urinary urgency and urinary frequency.

Past medical history: previous UTIs, congenital malformations, stone disease, immune-suppression. Get information from the prenatal ultrasound, like oligohydramnios. Drug history: immune-suppressants.

2. Physical examination: general condition, respiratory disorders, tachypnea, tachycardia, prolonged perfusion, hypotension, check for hydration, rule out testicular torsion and acute abdomen. Palpable bladder? Renal angle pain. Rule out phimosis or synechia of labia minora.

3. Investigations:
The objective is to electively rule out the unusual occurrence of obstruction, vesicoureteral reflux (VUR) and dysfunctional voiding. Should be triggered by two episodes of UTI in girls and one in boys.

Blood: FBC, culture if pyrexial. U&Es.

Imaging: USS if the UTI is severe, complicated or recurrent. VCU (voiding cystourethrography) electively if there is suspicion of reflux. DTPA/MAG3 diuretic renogram (electively for suspicion of dilatation/reflux).

Others: urine culture (the urine sample should be taken with supra pubic aspiration or catheterisation if it cannot be collected). Urine analysis (MSU). Dip for leucocytes and nitrates.

Treatment.
Medical.
Objectives are:
1. Elimination of symptoms and eradication of bacteriuria in the acute episode.
2. Prevention of renal scarring.
3. Prevention of recurrent UTIs.
4. Correction of associated urological lesions.
The scope of this book is to address point 1. The others should be done electively under the supervision of a specialist.

Severe UTI.
- Parenteral therapy until afebrile.
- Adequate hydration.
- Cephalosporins: Cephalexin 50-100 mg/kg TDS IV; Ceftriaxone IV 50-100 mg/kg OD. Amoxicillin/clavulanate if cocci are present: 60-100 mg/kg oral (37.5-75 mg/kg IV) TDS.

- All regimes followed by oral therapy to complete 10-14 days of treatment.

Simple UTI.
- Oral therapy: Cephalosporins.
- Parenteral single-dose therapy (only in case of doubtful compliance): Gentamicin 5mg/kg OD.
- Oral therapy to complete 5-7 days of treatment.

Surgical.
Drain any collections or abscess as in adults.

Complications.
The main long term complication is renal scarring and consequent renal failure, with or without hypertension. In the acute period take all measures to prevent sepsis and multi-organ failure.

Outcomes.
Very good if detected and treated early, and any underlying causes addressed.

Additional reading:
1. Paediatric urinary tract infections. Bhat RG, Katy TA, Place FC. Emerg Med Clin North Am. 2011 Aug; 29(3):637-53.
2. Paediatric urinary tract infections. Chang SL, Shortliffe LD. Pediatr Clin North Am. 2006 Jun; 53(3):379-400.
3. Urinary Tract Infection: Clinical Practice Guideline for the Diagnosis and Management of the Initial UTI in Febrile Infants and Children 2 to 24 Months. American Academy of Pediatrics. Pediatrics. 2011 Sep; 128(3): 595-610.
4. Urinary tract infection in under 16s: diagnosis and management. National Institute for health and Care Excellence (NICE). https://www.nice.org.uk/guidance/cg54/chapter/1-Guidance. On 20/03/2016.
5. Paediatric urinary tract infections. American Urological Association. https://www.auanet.org/education/pediatric-urinary-tract-infections.cfm. On 20/03/2016.
6. Diagnosis and Treatment of Urinary Tract Infections in Children. White B. Am Fam Physician. 2011 Feb 15; 83(4): 409-415.

1.6. Urosepsis.

Mr J Clavijo.

Definition.
It is sepsis due to an infection of the urogenital tract. Adult urosepsis comprises approximately 25% of all cases of sepsis, and it is in most cases secondary to complicated infections. Severe sepsis and septic shock are critical situations, with a mortality rate of 30% to 40%.

Aetiology.
Urosepsis is usually the result of an obstructive pyelonephritis with ureter stones being the most common cause. In this scenario an infection can rapidly develop into systemic multi-organ failure. Gram-negative bacteria are found in 70% of cases. Any cause of immunosuppression accelerates this process and makes it difficult to treat. Other common urogenital foci include: prostatitis, epididymo-orchitis and Fournier's gangrene.

Classification.
- Infection: a pathologic process caused by the invasion of normally sterile tissue or fluid by pathogenic or potentially pathogenic microorganisms.
- Sepsis: the presence of infection, documented or strongly suspected, with a systemic inflammatory response, as indicated by the presence of some of the systemic symptoms and signs.
- Severe sepsis: sepsis complicated by organ dysfunction.
- Septic shock: severe sepsis complicated by acute circulatory failure characterized by persistent arterial hypotension, despite adequate volume resuscitation, and unexplained by other causes.

Diagnosis.
Make an early working diagnosis, even if it is temporary.

1. History: rigor, fever (rarely hypothermia), symptoms of shock (tachycardia, tachypnea, hypotension, drowsiness or coma), location of focus or foci.
Background: genitourinary conditions. Recent instrumentation. Any cause of immune-suppression (diabetes, etc.). Medications: antibiotics (for resistance), corticosteroids, chemotherapy.

SIRS and Sepsis Definition (ACCP/SCCM-criteria)

SIRS Systemic Inflammatory Response Syndrome	2 or more of the following criteria: · Temperature > 38 °C or 36 °C · Heart rate > 90 beats/min · Respiratory rate > 20 breaths/min or PaCO 2 < 32 torr (< 4.3 kPa) · WBC > 12000 cells/mm 3, < 4000 cells/mm3, or > 10% immature(band) forms
Sepsis	Documented infection together with 2 or more SIRS criteria
Severe Sepsis	Sepsis associated with organ dysfunction, including, but not limited to, lactic acidosis, oliguria, hypoxemia, coagulation disorders, or an acute alteration in mental status
Septic Shock	Sepsis with hypotension, despite adequate fluid resuscitation, along with the presence of perfusion abnormalities. Patients who are on inotropic or vasopressor agents may not be hypotensive at the time when perfusion abnormalities are detected.

Severity	Gradient of severity →				
Symptoms	No symptoms	Local symptoms Dysuria, frequency, urgency, pain or bladder tenderness	+ General symptoms Fever, Flank pain Nausea, vomiting	Systemic response SIRS Fever, shivering Circulatory failure	Systemic response SIRS Organ dysfunction Organ failure
Diagnosis	ABU	CY-1	PN-2	PN-3 Febrile UTI	US-4	US-5	US-6
Investigations	Dipstick (MSU Culture + S as required)		Dipstick MSU Culture + S Renal US or I.V. Pyelogram /renal CT		Dipstick MSU Culture + S and Blood culture Renal US and/or Renal and abdominal CT
Risk factors	Risk factor assessment according to ORENUC (Table 2.1) →				
	Uncomplicated UTI		Complicated UTI		
Medical and surgical treatment	NO*	Empirical 3-5 days	Empirical + directed 7-14 days	Empirical + directed 7-14 days Consider combining 2 antibiotics	Empirical + directed 10-14 days Combine 2 antibiotics
				Drainage/surgery is required →	

EAU classification of UTIs.

Type	Category of risk factor	Examples of risk factors
O	No known/associated RF	- Healthy premenopausal women
R	RF of recurrent UTI, but no risk of severe outcome	- Sexual behaviour and contraceptive devices - Hormonal deficiency in post menopause - Secretory type of certain blood groups - Controlled diabetes mellitus
E	Extra-urogenital RF, with risk or more severe outcome	- Pregnancy - Male gender - Badly controlled diabetes mellitus - Relevant immunosuppression* - Connective tissue diseases* - Prematurity, new-born
N	Nephropathic disease, with risk of more severe outcome	- Relevant renal insufficiency* - Polycystic nephropathy
U	Urological RF, with risk or more severe outcome, which can be resolved during therapy	- Ureteral obstruction (i.e. stone, stricture) - Transient short-term urinary tract catheter - Asymptomatic Bacteriuria** - Controlled neurogenic bladder dysfunction - Urological surgery
C	Permanent urinary Catheter and non resolvable urological RF, with risk of more severe outcome	- Long-term urinary tract catheter treatment - Non-resolvable urinary obstruction - Badly controlled neurogenic bladder

UTI risk factors.[1]

2. Physical exam: look for foci on external genitalia. DRE: avoid "massaging" the prostate if infected (it produces bacteraemia). Oedema, positive fluid balance. Hypotension. Increased cardiac output . Pallor. Reduced urine output.

3. Investigations:
Blood: blood cultures, FBC (WCC, thrombocytopenia), ESR, procalcitonin and CRP. Kidney and liver function, hyperglycaemia. AB Gases (hypoxia, respiratory alkalosis or metabolic acidosis). Coagulation screen (DIC).

Imaging: the standard is contrast-enhanced CT if renal function is normal.

Treatment.
In an unstable patient, apply local trauma protocol/ATLS/ resuscitation immediately. Extensive monitoring. Use of inotropics and fluids as needed. Concomitantly give intravenous empirical antibiotics in high doses. Consider a beta-lactam (Amoxicillin) associated with aminoglycosides (Gentamicin) or alternatively a 3rd generation cephalosporin (Ceftriaxone). Be sure to achieve an optimal

oxygenation (saturation).

Surgical.
Once the patient is able to tolerate anaesthesia, drain the focus. This seems simple and intuitive but is a complex area, where there may be several options. Always drain pus and always drain an obstructed and infected system. Do it as soon as possible. If the patient is unstable and a high anaesthetic risk, use local anaesthesia and suitable needles or trocars to punction and drain. Once the patient is stable perform the most efficient operation for the case. These patients are more likely to survive if they are managed in intensive care by a multidisciplinary team. Discuss with all members immediate and medium-term plans. Run the plan without delay or hesitation. Remember that several operations may be necessary at the most appropriate times to achieve the best results.

Complications.
Septic shock, multiple organ failure and death. Recurrence of successive focus or foci. Progression of cellulitis. Antibiotic resistance.

Outcomes.
They depend on the balance between foci removal + antibiotics + multiple organ support, versus virulence + patient's immune response.

Additional reading:
1. Urinary tract infection. Nicolle LE. Crit Care Clin. 2013 Jul; 29(3): 699-715.
2. Diagnosis and management for urosepsis. Wagenlehner FM, Lichtenstern C, Rolfes C, Mayer K, Uhle F, Weidner W, Weigand MA.. Int J Urol. 2013 Oct; 20(10): 963-70.
3. 2001 SCCM/ESICM/ACCP/ATS/SIS International Sepsis Definitions Conference. Levy MM, Fink MP, Marshall JC, Abraham E, Angus D, Cook D, et al. Crit Care Med. 2003; 31(4): 1250-1256.
4. Urinary tract infections in adults. National Institute for health and Care Excellence (NICE). https://www.nice.org.uk/guidance/qs90. On 20/03/2016.
5. Adult UTIs. American Urological Association. https://www.auanet.org/common/pdf/education/Adult-UTI.pdf. On 20/03/2016.
6. Urological Infections. European Association of Urology Guidelines. http://uroweb.org/wp-content/uploads/EAU-Guidelines-Urological-Infections-v2.pdf. On 20/03/2016.
7. Sepsis and Non-infectious Systemic Inflammation. Edited by J.-M. Cavaillon and C. Adrie. 2009 WILEY-VCH Verlag GmbH & Co. KGaA, Weinheim. ISBN: 978-3-527-31935-0.

CHAPTER 2. Obstruction.

2.1. Acute urinary retention.

Mr S Salloum, Dr T Jora, Dr E Zungri and Mr J Clavijo.

Definition.
Urinary retention is the inability to voluntarily void some or all the urine in the bladder.

Aetiology.
- Increased urethral resistance (bladder outlet obstruction).
- Reduced bladder pressure (detrusor failure, spinal shock).
- A combination of the above.

Selected Causes of Urinary Retention:

Cause	Male	Female	Both
Obstructive	Benign prostatic hyperplasia; meatal stenosis; paraphimosis; pinhole phimosis; prostate cancer	Organ prolapse (cystocele, rectocele, uterine prolapse); pelvic mass (gynaecologic malignancy, uterine fibroid, ovarian cyst); retroverted impacted gravid uterus	Bladder calculi; bladder neoplasm; faecal impaction; gastrointestinal or retroperitoneal malignancy/mass; urethral strictures, foreign bodies in bladder, urethral stones
Infectious and inflammatory	Balanitis; prostatic abscess; prostatitis	Acute vulvo-vaginitis; vaginal lichen planus; vaginal lichen sclerosus; vaginal pemphigus; atrophic vaginitis	Bilharziasis; cystitis; echinococcosis; Guillain-Barré syndrome; herpes simplex virus; Lyme disease; peri-urethral abscess; transverse myelitis; tuberculosis cystitis; urethritis; varicella-zoster virus

| Other | Penile trauma, fracture, or laceration | Postpartum complication; urethral sphincter dysfunction (Fowler's syndrome) | Disruption of posterior urethra and bladder neck in pelvic trauma; postoperative complication; psychogenic (Hinman's syndrome); spinal shock; peripheral neuropathy; medication related |

Classification.

Acute urinary retention is the sudden and often painful inability to void despite having a full bladder.

Chronic urinary retention is painless retention associated with an increased volume of residual urine.

It can also be divided in neurogenic and non-neurogenic.

Diagnosis.

1. History: check previous lower urinary tract symptoms. Then predisposing factors: FH of prostate cancer, bladder stones, enlarged prostate, neurological insults. Trigger situations: use of diuretics, long journeys (hours without urination producing detrusor hiper-distention), food or alcoholic transgression, intense sexual activity, exposure to cold and other sympathetic autonomic stimuli, infection. Postoperative in general but more commonly in abdominal and pelvic operations.

Past medical history: operations and instrumentation of the urinary tract, co-morbidities. Previous episodes of retention. Drug history: medications, especially anti-cholinergics and anti-psychotics. Medications that can lead to retention:
   - Opioids and anaesthetics.
   - Alpha-adrenoceptor agonists.
   - Benzodiazepines.
   - Non-steroidal anti-inflammatory drugs.
   - Calcium-channel blockers.
   - Antihistamines.
   - Alcohol.

2. Physical examination: look for a full bladder (Fig. 2.1), phimosis, paraphimosis, meatal stenosis, organ prolapse (cystocele, rectocele, and uterine prolapse). DRE: prostate enlargement, prostate cancer, faecal impaction. Perform a neurological

assessment of pelvis and lower limbs to rule out spinal compromise or peripheral neuropathy.

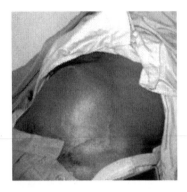

Fig. 2.1. Image shows lower abdominal distention in AUR.

3. Investigations:
Blood: FBC, U+E with eGFR, blood glucose, defer PSA (unless clinical suspicion of cancer).

Urine dip (when was it obtained): infection (leucocytes)?

Imaging:
USS of the bladder, prostate, and kidney for hydronephrosis, PVR (post void residual), and confirm AUR and its volume (which is usually done with an automated bladder scanner).

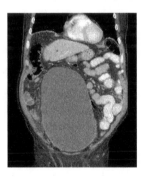

Fig. 2.2. CT shows distended bladder.

CT scan (Fig. 2.2) for any pelvic, abdominal, or retroperitoneal mass or malignancy causing extrinsic bladder neck compression, if suspected by the history/physical or other studies.

Other tests:
Cystoscopy if suspected bladder tumour and bladder or urethral stones or strictures.

Urodynamic studies to evaluate bladder function (elective).

Treatment.
Medical.
- Immediate decompression of the bladder through catheterization (See chapters on Urethral catheterisation and Suprapubic catheterisation). In cases of phimosis or paraphimosis, their treatment usually leads to urination.
- Document the PVR. Control urine output as it is possible to have **post-obstructive polyuria** where the urine output is very high and requires adequate fluid replacement. This should be detected in the first 3 to 6 hours after catheterisation, so observe the patient for this period. Use this time to check renal function and U&Es.
- Keep catheter for 3-7 days and prescribe Tamsulosin 400 mg OD at the time of catheterisation. Add 5-alpha reductase inhibitors like Finasteride 5mg OD in men with prostate enlargement by digital rectal examination.
- Trial without catheter (TWOC) in 3-7 days. Different protocols in different hospitals (check local protocol). Patients are able to void in 23-40% of cases and surgery, if needed, can be planned for a later date. Patients with PVR over 1 L will rarely resume voiding.
- Haematuria and hypotension are potential complications of rapid bladder decompression; drain the bladder slowly, particularly the first 100 ml (just place the collecting bag besides and at the level of the patient). **The discomfort of retention disappears after the first 50 ml or so are drained**. So, empty the rest of the bladder in 30 to 40 minutes.
- If the urethral catheterisation is impossible or contraindicated arrange for suprapubic catheter insertion. Intermittent self or assisted catheterisation is an alternative that can be considered.

Definitive management:
A urological consultation is paramount. Depending of the aetiology further treatment (elective) may involve surgical and/or medical manoeuvres. In case of BPH if the TWOC was unsuccessful consider TURP (transurethral resection of the prostate) or its surgical alternatives.
Hormonal treatment of advanced prostate cancer can lead to voiding in some scenarios.
For chronic urinary retention, especially in those with neurogenic

bladder, the first-line treatment is intermittent self-catheterization, as the complications of long term indwelling catheters include UTI, sepsis, trauma, stones, urethral strictures or erosions, prostatitis, and potential development of bladder squamous cell carcinoma.

Complications.
Acute renal failure, UTI, overflow incontinence, rarely intra-peritoneal bladder perforation.

Outcomes.
After catheterisation or supra-pubic drainage the outcome should be good in the short term. In the long term it will depend on the underlying aetiology and its treatment. The mortality rate associated with AUR increases considerably with age and comorbidity.

Additional reading:
1. EAU Guidelines on the Assessment of Non-neurogenic Male Lower Urinary Tract Symptoms including Benign Prostatic Obstruction. Gratzke C, Bachmann A, Descazeaud A, Drake J, Madersbacher S, Mamoulakis C, Oelke M, Tikkinen KA, Gravas S. Eur Urol. 2015 Jun; 67(6): 1099-109.
2. Urinary Retention in Adults: Diagnosis and Initial Management. Selius BA, R. Subedi R. Am Fam Physician, 2008, Mar 1; 77(5):643-650.
3. Acute urinary retention and urinary incontinence. Curtis LA, Dolan TS, Cespedes RD. Emerg Med Clin North Am. 2001; 19(3):600.
4. Management of obstructive voiding dysfunction. Ellerkmann RM, McBride A. Drugs Today (Barc). 2003; 39(7):515.
5. Lower urinary tract symptoms in men: management. National Institute for Health and Care Excellence. https://www.nice.org.uk/guidance/cg97/chapter/1-recommendations. On 22/03/2016.

2.2. Urethral catheter insertion.

Mr S Salloum, Sr S Larn and Dr E Zungri.

Definition.
It's the correct placement of a catheter in the bladder lumen through the urethra.

Introduction.
The ability to insert a urinary catheter is an essential basic skill in medicine. A Foley catheter (indwelling urinary catheter) is retained by means of a balloon at the tip that is inflated with sterile water. The balloons typically come in different sizes: 5, 10 and 30 ml. Catheters are commonly made in silicone rubber or natural rubber. Catheters are sized in units called French, where one French equals 1/3 of 1 mm. Catheters usually vary from 12 (small) Fr. to 24 (large) Fr. in size, according to stock policy (smaller and larger can be sourced on order). Catheters come in a variety of materials (latex, silicone, Teflon®) and types. These include Foley, straight catheter (Nelaton), Coudé tip catheter (hockey stick). Fig. 2.3.

Indications.
Acute indications include:
- Treatment of urinary retention.
- Preoperative prophylactic emptying of the bladder.
- Monitoring urine output in critically ill patients.
- Checking urinary residual volumes.
- Obtaining a urine specimen.
- Treatment of haematuria: to decompress the bladder and start the irrigation system (a 3 way large bore catheter should be inserted as a small one will be blocked with clots).
- Incontinence management in the short term.
- Postoperative bladder drainage and diuresis control.

In some cases, as in urethral strictures or prostatic hypertrophy, insertion will be difficult and early consultation with experienced members of the Urology team is essential.

Contraindications.
- Urethral injuries: urethral trauma may occur in patients with multi-system injuries and pelvic factures, as well as straddle

impacts. If this is suspected, one must perform a genital and rectal exam first. If one finds blood at the meatus of the urethra, a scrotal haematoma, a pelvic fracture, or a high riding prostate, there should be a high suspicion of urethral lesion. A retrograde urethrogram (injecting 20 ml of contrast into the urethra) must be obtained. If an injury is confirmed, open suprapubic catheter placement needs to be done.

- Urethritis and prostatitis (relative).

Technique.

Pre-procedural.

Patient informed about diagnosis and procedure with possible risks and complications and verbal consent obtained.

Prophylactic antibiotics administered if necessary. Prophylactic antibiotics are recommended for patients with prosthetic heart valves, artificial urethral sphincters, immunosuppression or penile prosthesis and when changing catheters with significant pyuria.

Prepare trolley: sterile pack with sterile drapes, antiseptic, sterile gloves, local anaesthetic, syringe with water to inflate balloon, urine bag. Catheters come with various tips. The standard straight is suitable for most cases. Tiemann or Coudé with a curved tip are designed to facilitate passage through the prostate, however they are better used by experienced team members. The whistle-tipped catheter has openings laterally and above the balloon to drain debris and clots.

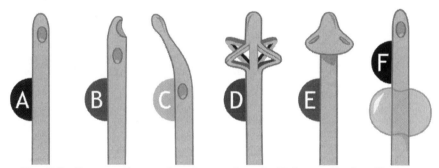

Fig. 2.3. Frequently used catheter tips. A. Nelaton. B. Coudé. C. Tiemann. D. Malecot. E. Pezzer. F. Foley.

Equipment:
- Sterile gloves.
- Sterile drapes.

- Cleansing solution (e.g. povidone, chlorhexidine or saline, depending on local protocol).
- Cotton swabs.
- Forceps.
- Sterile water (usually 10 cc).
- Foley catheter (usually 12-16 French) or 3 way Foley catheter in case of haematuria (18-22 Fr.).
- Syringe (usually 10-30 cc) depending on the catheter balloon's volume (written on the catheter).
- Lubricant (water based jelly or lidocaine gel 2%).
- Collection bag and tubing.

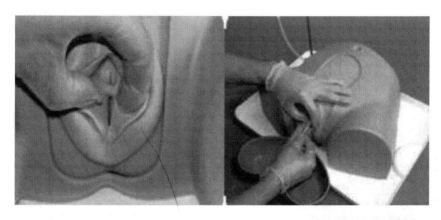

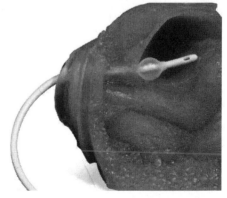

Fig. 2.4. Female catheterisation model.

Procedure.

Local protocols may vary slightly, so familiarise with your local one. Universal precautions: The potential for contact with a patient's body fluids while placing a catheter is present and increases with the inexperience of the operator. Gloves must be worn at all times. All team members should wear gloves, face and eye protection (optional) and gowns/apron.

1. Assist patient into supine position with knees extended in males and spread in females, and feet together.
2. Open catheterization kit and catheter.
3. Prepare sterile field, wear sterile gloves.
4. Check balloon for patency.
5. Generously coat the distal portion (2-5 cm) of the catheter with lubricant.
6. Apply sterile drape.
7. If female, separate labia using non-dominant hand (Fig. 2.4). If male, hold the penis with the non-dominant hand. Retract the prepuce. Maintain hand position until preparing to inflate balloon, use a dry swab around the base of the glans to assist you.
8. Use dominant hand to cleanse peri-urethral mucosa with cleansing solution. Cleanse anterior to posterior, inner to outer, one swipe per swab, discard swab away from sterile field.
9. Pick up catheter with gloved (and sterile) dominant hand.
10. In the male, lift the penis to a position perpendicular to patient's body and apply light upward traction (with non-dominant hand). Fig. 2.5.
11. Identify the urinary meatus and insert the anaesthetic lubricant (e.g. Instillagel®) 10 ml, wait for 2-3 min to let the local anaesthetic work.
12. Gently insert the catheter passing 1 to 2 inches beyond the point where urine is noted coming out of the catheter.
13. Inflate balloon, using correct amount of sterile liquid (usually 10 ml but check actual balloon size).
14. Gently pull catheter until inflated balloon is snug against bladder neck. Always pull the prepuce forward, failure to do so can cause a paraphimosis (iatrogenic).
15. Connect catheter to drainage system. Closed drainage system packs are now frequently available and help towards contamination control.
16. Secure catheter to abdomen or thigh, without tension on tubing.
17. Place drainage bag at or below level of bladder.
18. Evaluate catheter function and amount, colour, odour, and quality of urine.
19. Remove gloves, dispose of equipment appropriately, wash hands.
20. Document the size of the catheter inserted, amount of water in balloon, patient's response to procedure, and assessment of urine after the insertion of the catheter.

21. On the long term, the use of a catheter valve as an alternative to continuous free drainage should always be considered where the bladder is known to provide safe urinary storage.

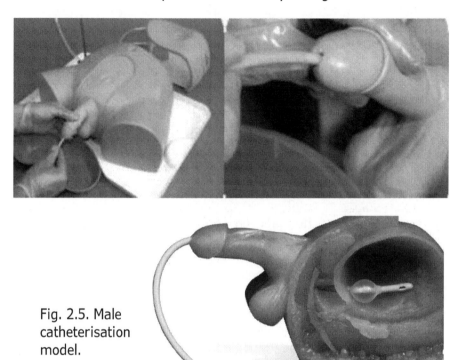

Fig. 2.5. Male catheterisation model.

Potential insertion difficulties:
- Phimosis: if the preputial opening is adequate, try to pass the catheter blind. If the opening is too narrow, try dilating it with sounds or a smaller catheter. If it fails, a preputial slit or circumcision may be needed (see Chapter 4.2).
- Failing to pass the prostate: try a catheter with a **larger** diameter. The prostatic urethra is not narrow but squashed flat by the surrounding prostate lobes. A larger catheter (harder to buckle) may overcome this problem. Another option is to try a silicone catheter, as it is more rigid than a latex one.
- Failing to pass the bladder neck: try a smaller size.
- False passage: higher risk, especially if catheterisation is traumatic. Never push past resistance during insertion. Opt for alternative drainage methods.
- Urinary retention: the lumen of the catheter may become blocked

(debris) if using too small bore catheter.

Complications.

- Inability to insert catheter which can cause urethral tissue trauma and bleeding to the point of false passage.
- Infection: prostatitis, pyelonephritis, cystitis, urosepsis. If there is an on-going infection give Gentamycin 3 mg/kg IV once prior to the procedure. With an indwelling catheter, bacteriuria becomes inevitable.
- Encrustation, stones.
- Bladder contractions around the balloon producing urgency, tenesmus, peri-catheter leak and pain. Try anticholinergics.
- Blockage requires catheter flushing or change.
- Urethral perforation. Traumatic hypospadias.
- Impossibility of catheter removal. We discuss here the case for Foley catheters. The main reason for the balloon not to deflate is malfunction of the inflation valve caused by its damage (crushing or twist). The valve can also be obstructed by crystallization when using fluids other than water to fill the balloon. Manoeuvres:

1. The first step is to cut the inflation valve off. This should allow the water to drain spontaneously. If this fails, the obstruction is in the inflation channel or at the entrance of the balloon.
2. The next manoeuvre is to advance a thin gauge metal guide wire (lubricated) through the filling channel. The guide or stylet must allow the fluid to drain around it.
3. If the above fails, a central venous catheter can be passed over the guide wire. When the catheter tip reaches the balloon, the guide can be removed, and the balloon should drain.
4. If the above techniques are unsuccessful, the balloon should be chemically dissolved. The literature mentions the use of ether, chloroform, acetone and mineral oil as some possible options. Mineral oil should be used as the other solutions are toxic to the bladder epithelium. Approximately 10 ml of mineral oil can be injected through the filling channel and the balloon will dissolve in about 15 minutes. If not, inject 10 ml more. In general, this technique has an 85-90% reported success rate. Do not over inflate the balloon with air or saline to try to burst it. This can cause severe pain and a ruptured bladder (if small).
5. If all the above has failed, the balloon should be punctured with a fine needle. In women, this can be done transurethral passing a lumbar needle by the side of the catheter after applying local

lidocaine. The puncture can also be done via the transvaginal route. In men the needle is introduced via the transabdominal (suprapubic), transperineal or transrectal approaches. This should always be done with the use of ultrasound guidance (Fig. 2.6 and Fig. 2.7) and preferably with a full bladder (fill through catheter with saline).

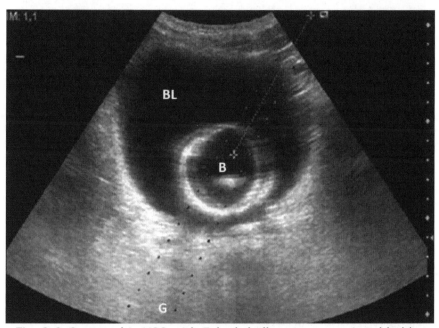

Fig. 2.6. Suprapubic USS with Foley's balloon snug against bladder neck (B), full bladder (BL), needle guide (G), and measurement of skin to balloon distance.

The alternatives to urethral catheterization include suprapubic catheterization, intermittent self (or assisted) catheterisation and external condom catheters (for continence).

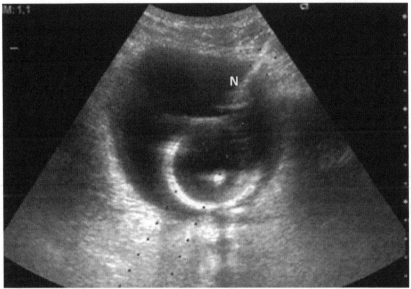

Fig. 2.7. Suprapubic USS with needle (N) advancing towards the balloon to be punctured.[2]

Additional reading:

1. How to manage a urinary catheter balloon that will not deflate. Patterson R, Little B, Tolan J, Sweeney C. Int Urol Nephrol. 2006; 38(1): 57-61.
2. Catheter valves: a welcome alternative to leg bags. Woodward S. Br J Nurs. 2013 Jun 13-26; 22(11):650, 652-4.
3. Urinary catheter policies for long-term bladder drainage. Niël-Weise BS, van den Broek PJ, da Silva EM, Silva LA. Cochrane Database Syst Rev. 2012 Aug 15; 8: CD004201.
4. Clinical and cost effectiveness of urethral catheterisation: a review. Scott BM. J Perioper Pract. 2010 Jul; 20(7): 235-40.
5. Impossible bladder catheter removal. What can we do? Molina Escudero R, Herranz Amo F, Lledo Garcia E, Husillos Alonso A, Ogaya Pinies G, Lopez Lopez E, Madrid Vallenilla A, Poza García A, Hernandez Fernandez C. Arch Esp Urol. 2012 May; 65(4): 489-92.
6. Guideline for Isolation Precautions: Preventing Transmission of Infectious Agents in Healthcare Settings. HICPAC. CDC. http://www.cdc.gov/hicpac/pdf/isolation/Isolation2007.pdf. On 21/03/2016.

2.3. Suprapubic catheter placement.

Mr S Salloum, Dr E Zungri and Mr J Clavijo.

Definition.
It is the placement of a catheter in the lower abdominal area that drains the bladder. In this chapter we will refer to the percutaneous insertion technique.

- Indications:
  1. Failed urethral catheterization in urinary retention.
  2. Urethral injury.
  3. Urethritis, prostatitis.

- Contraindications: absence of an easily palpable or ultrasound distended bladder. **It is critical and sometimes vital that the bladder is distended.** Bowel or vascular injuries are common when trying to puncture bladders with less than 200 mL inside.

- Relative contraindications:
  1. Clot retention, as there may be an underlying bladder cancer. Clots can rarely be cleared through a percutaneous SPC.
  2. Patients with hypogastric incisions (midline, Pfannenstiel).
  3. Pelvic fractures, which is an indication for open surgical SPC placement.
  4. Pelvic cancers.
  5. Coagulopathy producing haematuria.

Classification:
1. Seldinger technique: tract dilatation over a guide-wire. Fig. 2.8.

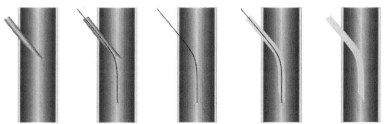

Fig. 2.8. Seldinger technique as initially described for vascular access.

2. Catheter over needle technique: one punction procedure with the catheter sequentially fitted around the needle. Fig. 2.9.

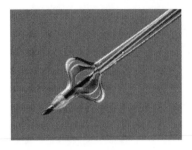

Fig. 2.9. Small Malecot catheter over needle.

3. Catheter through a trocar (Reuter's or Lawrence Add-a-Cath®). Fig. 2.10.

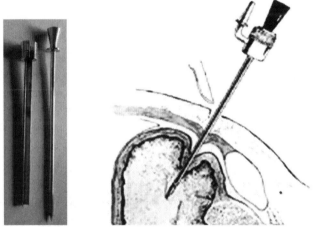

Fig. 2.10. Reuter's trocar and placement.

Technique.
Seldinger technique (over guide-wire) with a Foley catheter. There are several catheters that come in the kits and vary according to each manufacturer.

Procedure:

1. Abdominal examination (confirm that the bladder is distended). Fig. 2.11.
2. Have an USS or bladder scan to confirm a bladder volume of over 400 ml.
3. Patient informed about diagnosis and necessity of the procedure with possible risks and complications and verbal or written (preferably) consent obtained.

Fig. 2.11. Image:
Distended bladder on
examination.

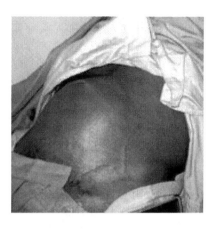

4. Universal precautions: the potential for contact with a patient's blood/body fluids while placing a SPC is present and increases with the inexperience of the operator. Gloves must be worn at all times. Trauma protocol calls for all team members to wear gloves, face and eye protection and gowns/apron.
5. Prepare trolley: sterile pack with sterile drapes, antiseptic, sterile gloves, local anaesthetic, syringe and needles, scalpel, sutures, suprapubic catheter, syringe with 10 ml water to inflate balloon, urine bag. Fig. 2.12

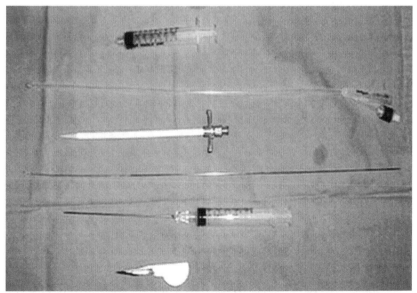

Fig. 2.12. SPC insertion kit (top to bottom): syringe, catheter, trocar/dilator with sheath, guide-wire, syringe with long needle, scalpel blade.

6. Prophylactic antibiotics administered if necessary.
7. Place the patient supine, in a moderate Trendelenburg position (head down) to facilitate the abdominal organs to move away from the pelvis by gravity.
8. Proceed with infiltration with local anaesthetic after antisepsis and draping. Do it 3-4 cm above symphysis pubis. Fig. 2.13.

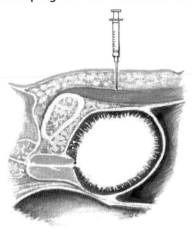

Fig. 2.13. Local anaesthetic before incision.

9. Incision: supra-pubic, midline, 1 cm, horizontal skin incision about 1-2 fingerbreadths above symphysis pubis using scalpel blade. Fig. 2.14.

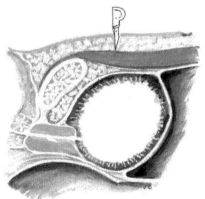

Fig. 2.14. Incision.

10. Confirmation of the intended tract going straight vertically at 90 degrees angle, with the long needle, and aspirating urine. Estimate approximate length of the tract from skin to the bladder. Perform an USS guided puncture if available, to try to avoid bowel

perforation. If in doubt, use a 27 or 30 G Chiba needle for aspiration. Fig. 2.15.

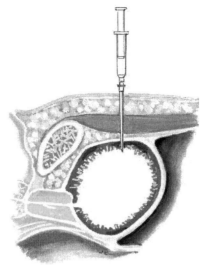

Fig. 2.15. Local anaesthetic and bladder aspiration with long needle.

11. Introduce a guide-wire with the floppy tip first, through the long needle into the bladder. Fig. 2.16.

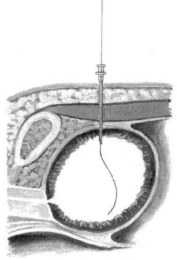

Fig. 2.16. Guide through long needle.

12. Remove needle, leaving the guide-wire in position, use non-dominant hand to **avoid guide displacement**. Dilate the tract by

advancing the trocar/dilator with its sheath over the guide-wire. Fig. 2.17.

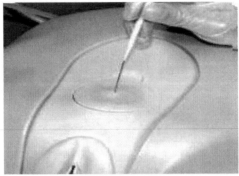

Fig. 2.17. Guide wire and tract dilatation in model.

13. The guide-wire can be removed once the trocar/dilator with its sheath is in the bladder (urine coming out).
14. The trocar/dilator only, is then rotated and removed, with the outer sheath left in place within the bladder lumen. **Avoid urine coming out and emptying the bladder** by occluding top of sheath with finger. Fig. 2.18.

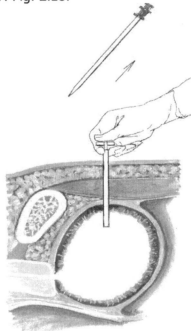

Fig. 2.18. Outer sheath left in place within the bladder.

15. A catheter (usually Foley) is inserted fully and the balloon inflated. The sheath can then be slid out and peeled apart for removal. Fig. 2.19 and 2.20.

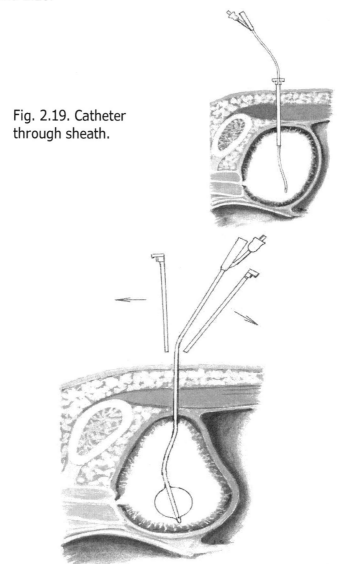

Fig. 2.19. Catheter through sheath.

Fig. 2.20. Catheter in place, sheath peeled apart, balloon inflated.

16. Urine bag attached, urine drained and volume recorded.
17. If any bleeding is present at the incision site, non-absorbable sutures may be needed to stop it and also to attach the catheter to the suprapubic skin preventing accidental removal (if balloon

fails).
18. Document procedure in patient's notes.
19. Arrange suprapubic catheter change in 6-8 weeks under skilled supervision. In the long term, the use of a catheter valve as an alternative to continuous free drainage should always be considered, where the bladder is known to provide safe urine storage. This prevents a small atrophic defunctionalized bladder.

Complications.
a) Visible haematuria is typically transient.
b) Post-obstruction increased diuresis is possible, and all patients should be observed for 3-6 hours. If this complication occurs, patients should be given intravenous fluids and correction of electrolytes (U&E).
c) Risk of cellulitis and abscess formation. Advice periodic wash and antiseptic clean.
d) Irrigation with saline should resolve most catheter obstructions. If displacement or wrong position is a concern, cystography should be performed.
e) Bowel perforation and intra-abdominal visceral or vascular injuries are possible. Ensure bladder distension with palpation and ultrasonography (or bladder scan) to minimize the chance of these complications. Sometimes ultrasound can also identify bowel loops in the working area.

Additional reading:
1. Suprapubic Foley Catheter Kit Executive Summary. NHS Technology Adoption Centre.
    http://webarchive.nationalarchives.gov.uk/20130701143131/http://www.ntac.nhs.uk/HowToWhyToGuides/SuprapubicFoleyCatheterKit/Catheter-Executive-Summary.aspx. On 01/07/2013.
2. British Association of Urological Surgeons' suprapubic catheter practice guidelines. Harrison SC, Lawrence WT, Morley R, Pearce I, Taylor J. BJU Int. 2011Jan; 107(1): 77-85.
3. Percutaneous Suprapubic Cystostomy. Satya Allaparthi; K. C. Balaji; Philip J. Ayvazian. In: Irwin and Rippe's Intensive Care Medicine, 7th Edition. Irwin, Richard S.; Rippe, James M. 2011. Lippincott Williams & Wilkins.
4. Guideline for Isolation Precautions: Preventing Transmission of Infectious Agents in Healthcare Settings. HICPAC. CDC. http://www.cdc.gov/hicpac/pdf/isolation/Isolation2007.pdf. On 21/03/2016.

2.4. Kidney colic.

Mr S Laghari, Mr P Verma and Professor A Rane.

Definition.
Genito-urinary pain can be due to obstruction of hollow organs, inflammation, distention of the capsule (e.g., kidney, prostate) or infiltration of adjacent nerves. Acute obstruction to hollow structures leads to colicky pain which is very severe. Obstruction that develops over a prolonged period will lead to dull ache (e.g. obstruction due to malignant disease). The pain experienced is mainly due to the increase in smooth muscle contraction of the ureter trying to overcome the obstruction. Since this contraction occurs in waves the pain experienced is also in periods. This smooth muscle contraction is mediated by prostaglandins.

Aetiology.
1. Calculus (lithiasis).
Stones commonly cause ureter obstruction at certain points of natural anatomical narrowing (Fig. 2.21):
   a) pelvic-ureteric junction,
   b) the level where the ureter crosses the iliac vessels (common iliac artery) and
   c) the vesico-ureteric junction.

Stones can be primary or secondary to other pathology, like pelvic-ureteric obstruction, mega-ureter, etc. In the latter patients apart from treating the stone the primary pathology must also be dealt with at some point.

2. Blood clots.
Haematuria and clot formation in the GU system can be due to stones, tumours, trauma, anti-coagulant treatment and vascular malformations. Tumours which cause bleeding can be malignant or benign. Malignant tumours can be renal parenchymal tumours like renal cell carcinoma, or urothelial tumours like transitional cell carcinoma. Benign tumours like angiomyolipomata can also cause haematuria.

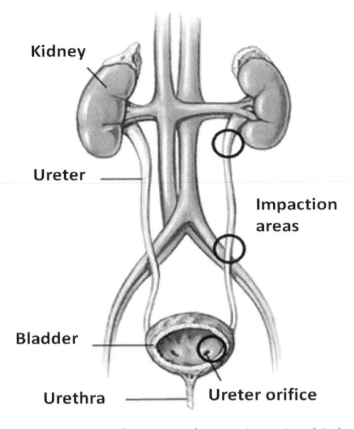

Fig. 2.21. Natural anatomical narrowing points (circles).

Trauma can occur due to blunt, penetrating or iatrogenic injuries (e.g. after biopsy, percutaneous procedures, etc.). More rarely vascular malformations like arterial-venous communication, aneurysm, and haemangiomas can all lead to bleeding and clot colic.

3. Necrosed papilla.
The renal papilla can lose its blood supply and subsequently necrotize and fall off causing obstruction. There are many causes for papillary necrosis like diabetes, analgesic abuse, sickle cell anaemia and infection to name a few.

4. Surgical ligation of ureter.
The common causes of accidental surgical ligation of the ureter are procedures like hysterectomy due to the close proximity of the distal ureter and the uterine artery.

Diagnosis.

1. History: severe colicky pain, vomiting, haematuria. The pain typically starts in the loin and radiates to the groin and iliac fossa. The pain can radiate to the labia/scrotum. Frequency, urgency and dysuria can happen in addition to colicky pain if the stone is close to the VUJ (vesical ureteric junction). Patients with infection can present with fever and chills. All patients presenting with loin pain, fever and chills must be suspected of having obstructive pyelonephritis (see chapter).

Differentials: patients with abdominal pain due to renal colic can sometimes be confused with intraperitoneal pathology. Patients with peritoneal inflammation will have guarding, rebound tenderness, rigidity and will prefer to stay still as movement will aggravate pain. Patients with renal colic will be rolling and there will not be signs of peritonitis. The pain of a dissecting aortic aneurism tends to be constant rather than colic.

Past medical history: previous stone disease or urological malignancy. Enquire about family history of stone disease. Drug history: chemotherapy, anti retrovirals, particularly Indinavir.

2. Physical examination: abdomen: rule out guarding. Palpable kidney, aorta?

3. Investigations:
Urine dip: look for blood, nitrates, and leucocytes. If leucocytes are present, then request urine culture and treat as coexistent infection.

Blood: FBC, U+E to check renal function. If the patient is septic, request blood culture. Calcaemia and uric acid. Uric acid.

Imaging: the imaging of choice is CT KUB (computed tomography of kidneys ureter and bladder) without contrast (Fig. 2.22) which should be done as soon as possible. The Hounsfield units reasonably predict stone response to shock wave lithotripsy (under 800 HU).

An X ray of the KUB area can also be used (Fig. 2.23). Radio opaque shadows can be seen in the renal area (useful for calcific stones, circa 80% overall).

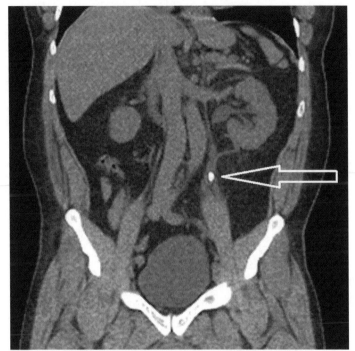

Fig. 2.22. CT KUB shows a stone in the left ureter (arrow).

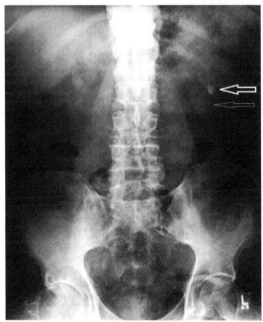

Fig. 2.23. This KUB demonstrates two radio-opaque renal calculi
projected over the lower pole of the left kidney (arrow).

Ultrasound: hydro/hydro-uretero -nephrosis, calculi, and renal masses can be detected. It is minimally invasive, does not use radiation and therefore can be repeated as needed. Fig. 2.24.

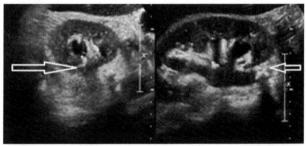

Fig. 2.24. USS of the right kidney shows a stone with distal shadow (arrows).

IVU: alternative if CT KUB is not available. The patient needs to have normal renal function as i/v contrast is used.

Treatment.
Patients who present with colic will need both symptomatic relief as well as definitive treatment of the obstruction.

Medical.
Conservative treatment is acceptable for stones <5 mm as they have a higher chance of spontaneous passage.
A. Symptomatic pain relief: Diclofenac 25-50 mg TDS, the mainstay of symptomatic relief. If it is not sufficient: Morphine 0.1 mg/Kg oral, I/V or I/M + antiemetic TDS/QDS.
B. Medical expulsion therapy: Tamsulosin 400 micrograms OD. This relaxes the smooth muscle of the ureter and enhances the chance of stone expulsion (~ 30%). If the stone is not expelled in 2 to 4 weeks, or pain is not controllable, then other treatment options must be considered. The patient should sieve the urine (paper coffee filters) and control the temperature during this period. A KUB +/- USS should be done as periodic follow up evaluation.

Surgical.
Emergency procedures.
Emergency de-obstruction should be considered in the following situations:
• Patients with signs of infection, as infection in the presence of obstruction can lead to sepsis, bacteraemia, multiple organ failure

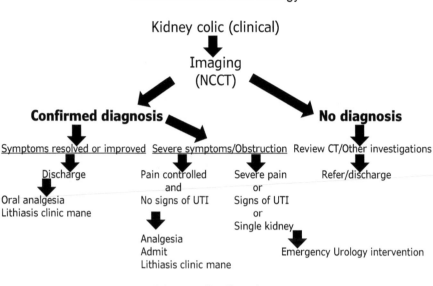

Kidney colic flowchart.

and death. It also produces rapid loss of function in the affected kidney.
- Severe pain not controlled by analgesics.
- Bilateral obstruction or obstruction of a single functioning kidney.

De-obstruction can be achieved by the following methods:
- **Percutaneous nephrostomy**: the main advantage is that it can be done under local anaesthesia and gives excellent decompression. The presence of pelvi-calyceal dilatation makes the procedure more likely to be successful.
- **Stenting**: most patients will need general anaesthesia, but can be done under local anaesthesia occasionally (females or with flexible cystoscope). If the obstruction is too tight (space between stone and ureter wall) then it might be difficult to bypass the stone in which case a nephrostomy has to be done.
- **Ureteroscopy** and lithotripsy (or litholapaxy) +/- stenting. The advantage of doing an ureteroscopy is that the primary pathology can be treated, resulting in decompression, most of the times. Ureteroscopy, like stenting, is preferably avoided in patients with infection as it may lead to increased retrograde intra luminal pressure and consequent retrograde haematogenous (systemic) spread of the infection.

Percutaneous nephrostomy.

A nephrostomy (Fig. 2.25) is a surgical procedure by which a tube, stent, or catheter is inserted through the skin and into the renal collecting system.

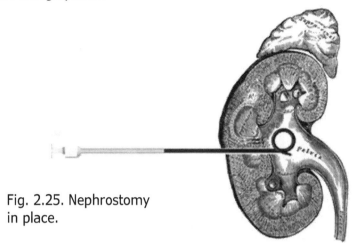

Fig. 2.25. Nephrostomy in place.

Indications:
- Treatment of urine blockage due to stone or tumour.
- Treatment of obstructive pyelonephritis.
- Access for interventions such as direct infusion of solutions for dissolving stones, chemotherapy, and antibiotic or antifungal therapy.
- Access for other procedures (e.g. benign stricture dilatation, antegrade ureteral stent placement, stone retrieval, pyelo-ureteroscopy, percutaneous nephro-lithotomy -PCNL- or endopyelotomy).
- Decompression of renal collections (e.g. abscesses).
- Treatment of urinary tract obstruction related to pregnancy.

Contraindications: bleeding diathesis (most commonly Warfarin, or uncontrollable coagulopathy), uncooperative patient, severe hyper-kalemia (>7 mEq/L); this should be corrected with haemodialysis before the procedure.

Preparation: coagulation screen and antibacterial prophylactics.

Technique:

Universal precautions: the potential for contact with a patient's blood/body fluids is present and increases with the inexperience of the surgeon. All team members to wear gloves, face and eye protection and gowns/apron if the procedure is done outside operating theatres (e.g. Radiology suite). Under local or general anaesthesia a very thin needle (Chiba) is inserted into the kidney with anatomical, USS or CT scan guidance. Usually with the patient in ventral decubitus (prone). Through this needle, aspiration of urine for culture can be obtained. Later, contrast is injected slowly. This allows for C arm radiological control of the whole procedure. Then a slightly larger needle is advanced through the external lateral side of the kidney, into the selected calyx. Then, a fine guide-wire follows through the needle. The needle is withdrawn and the guide-wire left into the collecting system. The catheter, which is about the same diameter as an I/V (intravenous) cannula, follows over the guide-wire to its proper location (Seldinger method). The catheter is then connected to a bag outside the body that collects the urine. The catheter and bag are secured so that the catheter will not pull out. Fig. 2.26.

Complications: bleeding (haematuria, peri renal haematoma), risk of bowel injury and intra-renal vascular lesion (arterio-venous fistula).

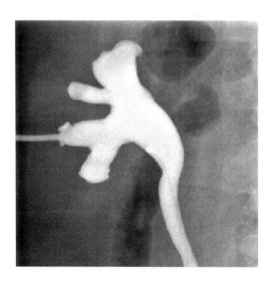

Fig. 2.26. Nephrostomy and contrast in the collecting system (antegrade nephrostogram).

JJ stent insertion.

A JJ stent placement (Fig. 2.27) is a surgical endoscopic procedure by which a tube (stent) is inserted through the bladder and the ureter meatus up and into the kidney by means of a cystoscope.

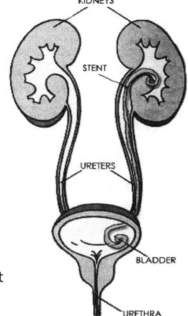

Fig. 2.27. JJ stent diagram.

Indications: to relieve upper urinary tract obstruction due to intrinsic (stone) or extrinsic compression.

Technique:
Usually in theatre and under general anaesthesia. After cystoscopy and defining the ureteral orifice of the obstructed kidney unit, an open-ended ureteral catheter is placed into the appropriate ureter meatus, so that a retrograde pyelogram (RPG) can be performed to delineate the anatomy of the collecting system as well as the point of obstruction. A guide-wire is then placed through the ureteral catheter, and the wire and catheter are navigated up into the desired kidney, bypassing the point of obstruction under fluoroscopic (X Ray) and cystoscopy guidance. The open ended ureteral catheter is removed. The JJ stent can be then placed over the guide-wire under a combination of cystoscopy and fluoroscopic guidance. The JJ stent is pushed over the wire till its distal end becomes flush with the cystoscope. A pusher is then advanced up to the JJ stent. The JJ stent

is then pushed up till the second and distal loop is at the ureter meatus (usually marked on the stent). Then the guide-wire is pulled out. The distal end of the stent can be seen coiling in the bladder, and the proximal one in the renal pelvis. Fig. 2.28.

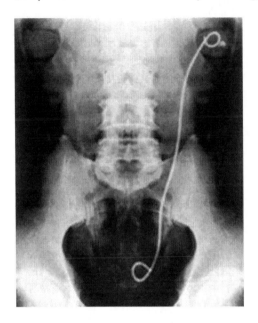

Fig. 2.28. X-ray showing normal position of the left stent.

Complications:
a) Ureteral or renal pelvic perforation.
b) Failure to bypass the obstruction.
c) Sepsis.

Elective procedures.
Once de-obstruction is achieved, subsequent treatment of the stone will be planned according to its composition, size and location(s). The various options include: Extracorporeal Shock Wave Lithotripsy (ESWL®, Fig. 2.29), ureteroscopy with or without stone fragmentation (Fig. 2.30), percutaneous nephrolithotomy (PCNL, for stones in the upper ureter and renal pelvis) and more rarely open or laparoscopic procedures (Fig. 2.31). The indications of each type of lithotripsy and fragmentation modalities are beyond the scope of this book, please see references for further reading.

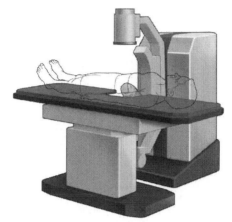

Fig. 2.29. Shock Wave Lithotripsy machine.

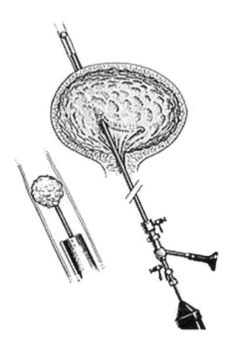

Fig. 2.30. Ureteroscopy with pneumatic lithotripter.

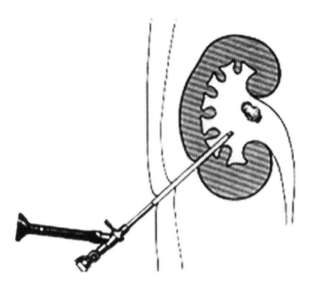

Fig. 2.31. Percutaneous nephrolithotomy.

Additional reading:

1. Diagnosis and management of renal (ureteric) colic. Ahmed HU, Khan AA, Bafaloukas N, Shergill IS, Buchholz NP. Br J Hosp Med (Lond). 2006 Sep; 67(9): 465-9.
2. Management of renal colic. Bultitude M, Rees J. BMJ. 2012 Aug 29; 345: e5499.
3. Suspected ureteral colic: plain film and sonography vs unenhanced helical CT. A prospective study in 66 patients. Ripollés T, Agramunt M, Errando J, Martínez MJ, Coronel B, Morales M. Eur Radiol. 2004 Jan; 14(1): 129-36.
4. Renal calculi: emergency department diagnosis and treatment. Carter MR, Green BR. Emerg Med Pract. 2011 Jul; 13(7): 1-17.
5. Guidelines for the acute management at first presentation of renal/ureteric lithiasis (excluding pregnancy). The British Association of Urological Surgeons. http://www.baus.org.uk/_userfiles/pages/files/Publications/RevisedAcuteStoneMgtGui delines.pdf. On 21/03/2016.
6. Management of ureteral calculi. EAU/AUA Nephrolithiasis Guideline Panel. https://www.auanet.org/education/guidelines/ureteral-calculi.cfm. On 21/03/2016.

2.5. Management of obstructive renal failure.

Mr P Verma and Mr J Clavijo.

Definition.
Obstructive renal failure is the loss of renal function secondary to an obstructive uropathy. Renal failure is also expletively referred to as "CKD" (chronic kidney disease).

Aetiology.
Obstruction to the flow of urine can cause changes in the renal system and if it results in bilateral obstruction they can cause renal failure. If the obstructive pathology is picked up early and appropriately treated then renal function can be restored and loss of nephrons can be minimized, a delay in the relief of obstruction will not normalize renal function.

Classification.
The causes of obstructive uropathy can be supravesical, vesical or infravesical. Supravesical pathologies have to be bilateral or obstruction of a single functioning kidney to produce a significant renal dysfunction, in severe cases this can present as anuria.

1. Supravesical causes (Fig. 2.32).
- Intraluminal: stones and clots.
- Mural: tumours of ureter/pelvis, bilateral PUJ obstruction, ureteric strictures (e.g. post radiotherapy or instrumentation).
- Extramural: retroperitoneal fibrosis (primary/secondary), lymph node compression of ureters, AAA, large infiltrating pelvic tumours.

2. Vesical causes.
- High pressure bladder with bilateral reflux.
- Large bladder tumour.
- Gross cystocele causing ureteric kinking and obstruction.

3. Infravesical causes.
- Enlarged prostate causing high pressure voiding or retention.

- Stricture of urethra.
- Severe phimosis (pinhole).

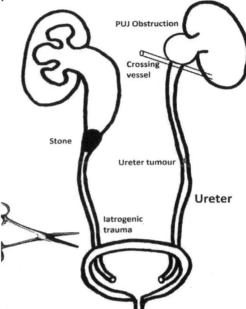

Fig. 2.32. Some causes of obstruction of the ureter.

Diagnosis

1. History: the clinical features can vary depending on what causes the obstruction. Features of renal failure (uraemia) such as nausea, vomiting and fluid retention can be present. The renal inability to clear waste may lead to complications, including metabolic acidosis, high potassium, and changes in fluid balance. Can be asymptomatic.

Past medical history: personal and family history of nephro-urological disease (stones). Radiotherapy, AAA. Drug history: nephrotoxic medication including: chemotherapy, aminoglycosides, NSAIDs, angiotensin-converting enzyme (ACE) inhibitors, i/v contrast.

2. Physical examination: hydration, cardiovascular, temperature. Full abdominal, pelvis and genital. Palpable abdominal masses, prostate, genital prolapse.

3. Investigations.

Blood: renal function tests must be done in all patients along with electrolytes as there can be gross changes in electrolytes which if not corrected appropriately can be life threatening. In the extremes of life (children and elderly) use clearance methods, as eGFR is less accurate. ABGs looking for metabolic acidosis. Cultures (blood, urine) if temperature.

Imaging: various radiological investigations can be used to diagnose the cause of the obstruction. Depending on the clinical suspicion and renal function one of the following can be used:
a) Ultrasound.
b) CT scan (without contrast if renal function is altered). Fig. 2.33.

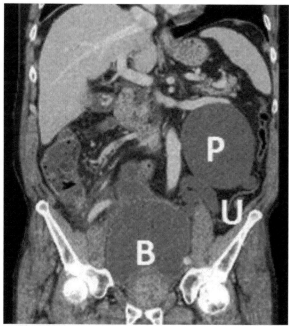

Fig. 2.33. CT shows dilatation of bladder (B), left ureter (U) and renal pelvis (P) secondary to infra-vesical obstruction.

c) MRI (without contrast if renal function is altered).

Others:
•   ECG: evidence of hyperkalaemia.
•   Urine dip and test. Culture if infection is suspected.

Treatment.
Surgical.
The main idea when treating these patients is to save the kidney(s) function and also treat the underlying pathology. To save kidney

function, the urinary tract should be de-obstructed at the earliest and this depends on the level of obstruction.

If the level of obstruction is supravesical the options are[3]:
1. Double J stent placement.
2. Percutaneous nephrostomy.
Uni- or bilateral depending on the situation.

If the obstruction is vesical or infravesical:
1. Urethral catheterization.
2. Suprapubic cystostomy (to be avoided if bladder tumour is suspected).

Once the obstruction is by passed then definitive treatment can be electively planned for the primary pathology (obstructive cause).

Medical.
Correct volume alterations. Stop and treat aggravating factors.
Post de-obstruction reactive increased diuresis should be anticipated. Patients can pass large quantities of urine which is diluted and if volume is not adequately replaced, it can push them into dehydration and hypotension. Most patients would need intravenous fluids. The causes of this diuresis are:
a) Impaired sodium reabsorption.
b) Impaired urine concentrating ability.
c) Solute diuresis (retained urea being eliminated).
d) Decreased responsiveness to ADH.

Contact a medical or nephrology team for their input. Renal failure is not a urological condition and these patients are better served by a strict nephrology control. Renal function replacement therapy may be needed. Methods of renal replacement therapy include: intermittent haemodialysis (IHD), continuous veno-venous hemodiafiltration (CVVHD), and peritoneal dialysis (PD). Each has advantages and limitations.

Complications.
Obstruction of the urinary tract will progressively destroy glomeruli, and consequently result in reduced renal function to the point of end

---

[3] Both are described in the kidney colic chapter (2.4).

stage renal failure. This requires renal replacement treatment which has significant cost, morbidity and mortality. If infected, obstruction can easily and rapidly progress to sepsis and death.

Outcomes.

It will depend on the kidneys' recovery capacity and the duration of the insult. The presence of infection considerably accelerates the deterioration of renal function.

Additional reading:

1. Chronic kidney disease in kidney stone formers. Rule AD, Krambeck AE, Lieske JC. Clin J Am Soc Nephrol. 2011 Aug; 6(8): 2069-75.
2. Anuria secondary to peri-aneurysmal fibrosis. Vallejo Gil C, García Rojo D, Banús Gassol JM, Fernández V, Muniesa Caldero M, Soler Roselló A. Actas Urol Esp. 1994 Jul-Aug; 18(7): 758-60.
3. Acute kidney injury in the elderly: a review. Chronopoulos A, Rosner MH, Cruz DN, Ronco C. Contrib Nephrol. 2010; 165: 315-21.
4. A framework and key research questions in AKI diagnosis and staging in different environments. Murray PT, Devarajan P, Levey AS, Eckardt KU, Bonventre JV, Lombardi R, Herget-Rosenthal S, Levin A. Clin J Am Soc Nephrol. 2008 May; 3(3): 864-8.
5. Obstructive acute renal failure by a gravid uterus: a case report and review. Brandes JC, Fritsche C. Am J Kidney Dis. 1991 Sep; 18(3): 398-401.

CHAPTER 3. Haematuria.

Mr M Rogers, Mr S Salloum, Dr R Molina and Mr J Clavijo.

"Nature shows us only the tail of the lion."
Albert Einstein. 1914.

Definition.
It is the presence of red blood cells (RBC) in the urine. It can be highly suspected by dipstick test (shows presence of Hem molecule) and confirmed by microscopy (> 3 RBC per HPF). It can also be seen (> 100 RBC per HPF) in case of frank haematuria (or clots) and that is diagnostic.

Aetiology.
The fact that the presence of RBCs in the urine can be physiologic explains why a substantial proportion of patients with microscopic and dipstick haematuria, and even macroscopic one, will have normal investigations. No abnormality is found in approximately 40% of subjects with macroscopic (visible) and 80% with microscopic haematuria (non visible), despite full conventional urological investigations (urine cytology, cystoscopy, CT scan, USS, and/or IVU). The most frequent pathological causes include UTIs, urothelial tumours, urinary tract stones, benign prostatic hypertrophy and prostate cancer.

Classification.
There are different kinds of classifications.
1. According to anatomical localisation:
a) Pre renal: hypertensive nephropathy, chronic heart failure, leukaemia, purpura, thrombocytopenia, excessive anticoagulation, haemophilia, sickle cell disease. Vascular: arterio-venous malformation, arterial emboli or thrombosis, arterio-venous fistula, renal vein thrombosis.
b) Renal: papillary necrosis, IgA nephropathy, posts streptococcal GN, interstitial nephritis, haemolytic-uremic syndrome, infections (pyelonephritis, TB, etc.). Connective tissue disease: Wegener's, Goodpasture's syndrome, HSP. Urological causes: trauma to any part of the urinary system, stones, arterio-venous malformations, nutcracker syndrome (compression of the left renal vein between

the aorta and the superior mesenteric artery), malignancy (renal cell carcinoma, Wilm's tumour, renal pelvis TCC), polycystic kidney, renal infarcts.

c) Post renal: ureter malignancy, stricture, stone, and papilloma. Bladder/prostate: BPH, malignancy (TCC, prostate cancer), stones, cystitis, prostatitis, polyps, schistosomiasis. Urethra: injury, urethritis, calculi, papilloma, ulcers on meatus.

2. According to symptoms:
- Visible. Frank or macroscopic. Non Visible. Microscopic haematuria: >3 red blood cells per high power field.
- False + Dipstick: myoglobinuria, bacterial peroxidases, hypochlorite, iodine disinfectants. False – Dipstick: RBC in presence of reducing agents (ascorbic acid).

Diagnosis.
1. History: full urological. Strenuous exercise, trauma.
Past medical history: stones, personal and family nephro-urological conditions, operations. Drug history: Rifampicin, Nitrofurantoin, Senna, Phenazopyridine, L- dopa, Metronidazole, Anticoagulants, Anti-platelets.

2. Physical examination: abdominal masses, blood pressure, full pelvic and genital (Fig. 3.1).

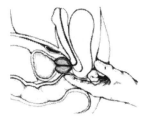

Fig. 3.1. DRE: prostate enlargement or cancer. Palpable bladder mass.

3. Investigations.
Imaging: upper urinary tract evaluation: CT scan (Fig. 3.2). If unavailable, MRI, USS or IVU.

Others:
Lower urinary tract evaluation by cystoscopy (Fig. 3.3). Elective if possible.

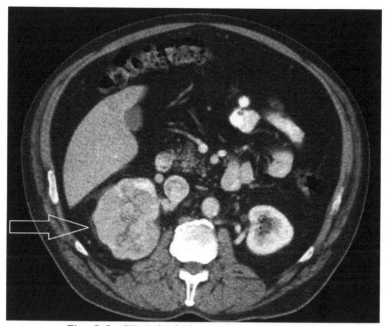

Fig. 3.2. CT right kidney tumour (arrow).

Urine cytology or urine tumour markers (BTA, NMP22).
Urine dipstick (UTI, proteinuria) and urine test including microscopic analysis. Fig. 3.4.

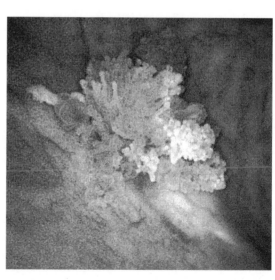

Fig. 3.3. Cystoscopy: bladder cancer above right ureteric orifice.

Blood: PSA, renal function, FBC, coagulation screen, blood group and cross match (in hypotensive patients).

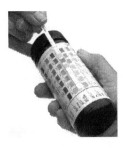

Fig. 3.4. Urine dip-stick
test, for Hem.

All patients with haematuria in absence of infection should be studied according to local protocol. It does not need to be urgent.

Elective nephrology referral for: patients who had a urological cause excluded, evidence of declining GFR, Stage 4 or 5 CKD (eGFR <30ml/min), proteinuria, haematuria with hypertension in younger than 40 years, haematuria with intercurrent (usually upper respiratory tract) infection, patient less than 16 years old.

Differentials:
• Haemoglobinuria: dipstick-positive (Hem), but no red cells on microscopy. Look for haemolysis.
• Myoglobinuria: dipstick-positive (Hem), but no red cells on microscopy. Look for myolysis (trauma, etc.).
• Food, (e.g. beetroot) and colorants. Dipstick negative.
• Drugs, e.g. Rifampicin, Nitrofurantoin, Senna. Dipstick negative.
• Porphyria: urine darkens on standing. Dipstick negative.
• Bilirubinuria: obstructive biliary disease. Bilirubin on dipstick.

Treatment.
Resuscitate with IV fluids/blood if in shock.

Continuous bladder irrigation: insert wide bore (>20 Fr) 3 way Foley catheter + continuous saline irrigation (alternative: bladder wash out) till the bleeding stops, clots are removed and the irrigation comes out reasonably clear. Apply intermittent catheter traction if needed (20 min on/off), this will compress the prostate and may reduce prostate related bleeding. Fig. 3.5.

If the bleeding doesn't stop, producing recurrent hypotension or requiring repeated transfusions, an emergency intervention is likely required: cystoscopy and bladder evacuation of clots and haematuria, +/- coagulation, TURBT/TURP. It is an exploratory endoscopy proceeding to a haemostatic operation according to the findings.

If the intra-haemorrhagic cystoscopy shows that it is an upper tract bleeding, the patient will require an emergency angiogram and embolization (renal or segmental) or nephrectomy (if patient remains unstable).

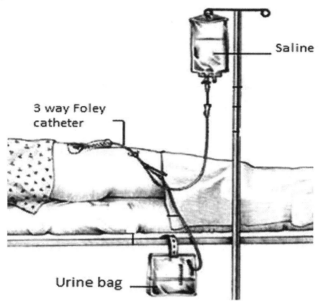

Fig. 3.5. Continuous bladder irrigation setup.

Elective: mild macroscopic and asymptomatic microscopic haematuria need outpatient Urology referral, and investigations and treatment depending of the cause.

Complications.
They will depend on the haemodynamic consequences of the bleeding. Outcomes will depend on the aetiology and treatment of the underlying pathology.

Additional reading:
1. Joint Consensus Statement on the Initial Assessment of Haematuria. The British Association of Urological Surgeons. http://www.baus.org.uk/professionals/baus_business/publications/17/haematuria_guide lines. On 21/03/2016.
2. In search of a consensus: evaluation of the patient with haematuria in an era of cost containment. Heller MT, Tublin ME. AJR Am J Roentgenol. 2014 Jun; 202(6): 1179-86.
3. Assessment of haematuria. Margulis V, Sagalowsky AI. Med Clin North Am. 2011

Jan; 95(1): 153-9.

4. Haematuria: etiology and evaluation for the primary care physician. Patel JV, Chambers CV, Gomella LG. Can J Urol. 2008 Aug; 15 Suppl 1: 54-61.

5. Haematuria. American Urological Association. https://www.auanet.org/education/hematuria.cfm. On 21/03/2016.

6. Urinary markers in screening patients with haematuria. Chiong E, Gaston KE, Grossman HB. World J Urol. 2008 Feb; 26(1): 25-30.

7. Long-term outcome of home dipstick testing for haematuria. Madeb R, Messing EM. World J Urol. 2008 Feb; 26(1): 19-24.

CHAPTER 4. External Genital Emergencies.

4.1. Acute scrotal pain.

Mr T Rosenbaum, Dr T Jora and Mr J Clavijo.

Definition.
Pain developed in the last 24 hours in the scrotum. It can also be intermittent or with previous episodes.

Aetiology.
Scrotal causes of acute pain:
1. Testicular torsion: a twist in the spermatic cord resulting in circumferential occlusion of the spermatic artery leading to interruption of the blood supply to the testis. The testis is consequently lying higher in the scrotum towards the inguinal canal. It produces ischaemia and gangrene unless corrected immediately. The torsion can be at various levels depending on the anatomy. The vascular occlusion is often progressive and tightens with the oedema. Sudden, severe acute pain, swelling and retraction. Occurs at any age but most common and relevant in children and young adults. Very relevant but difficult to diagnose in infants. The most common presentation is: acute pain, acute scrotal tumour without temperature.

2. Acute Epididymo-orchitis: inflammation of the spermatic cord, epididymis and the testis (see urinary infections chapter). It is rarely of sudden onset. Can also be chronic. Can be associated to a UTI, STD and to urethral catheters. The most common presentation is: progressive pain, progressive swelling, redness, warmer testis (inflammation) and pyrexia.

3. Torsion of the Appendix Testis (Hydatid of Morgagni) and/or the Appendix Epididymis: again this is a sudden onset of unilateral scrotal pain. However in this case there is tenderness at the upper pole of the testis, and the testicle usually hangs normally in the scrotum. The pain is less severe and is typically localised to a small area over the testis. Sometimes a small darkened area can be seen through the skin. The most common presentation is: acute pain in the upper pole of testis, small acute scrotal tumour in that area without temperature.

4. Haematocele: following trauma or scrotal surgery (e.g.

vasectomy). Testicular rupture: also usually caused by trauma and produces important hematoma (see trauma chapter). The most common presentation is: acute pain, acute scrotal tumour without temperature after trauma or surgery.

5. Testicular haematoma: usually due to trauma. Sub-albuginea haematoma can produce severe pain and lead to pressure ischemia (see trauma chapter). Haemorrhage or ischaemia of a testicular tumour: more common in fast growing tumours. Important to recognise as surgery via the scrotum should be avoided. Acute pain in a pre-existing tumour is an important, though rare, complication of testicular tumours. The swelling exposes the testes to trauma; fast growth can become ischaemic and bleed. On examination the size of the scrotal swelling is much larger than expected and a shy young adult may admit to having noted the increasing swelling for some time. Do not explore via de scrotum as this risks neoplastic contamination of inguinal lymphatics. Document your suspicion and confirm by ultrasound scan.

Referred causes of scrotal pain:
1. Strangulated hernia, inguinal or femoral: tender, painful, inguinal lump. It may present as intestinal obstruction or abdominal pain. In case of indirect inguinal hernia, there is an upper scrotal mass. A scrotal swelling which you cannot get your fingers above is a hernia unless proven otherwise. If it also hurts it can be an incarcerated hernia which may contain omentum, bowel or bladder. This may or may not be strangulated. Refer promptly to general surgery.

2. Appendicitis: the appendix shares the same visceral afferent nerve supply (T10) as the testes and this can cause referred pain. Scrotal examination will be normal.

3. Ureteric stone or any obstruction of the ureter: produces pain radiating to the groin, again of similar afferent pathway. Scrotal examination will be normal.

A. Testicular torsion.
Normal testicular fixation to the posterior part of the tunica vaginalis prevents twisting of the cord. The bell clapper deformity or lack of

fixation posteriorly, results in the testes being free to move within the tunica vaginalis virtual cavity. Contraction of the cord muscles (cremaster) shortens the spermatic cord and can produce testicular torsion (as the cremaster spirals down the cord). The degree of torsion varies from ½ to 2 loops of the cord. Increasing oedema reduces even more the testis blood supply.

Diagnosis.

A suspected testicular torsion is a clinical diagnosis. There is no place for any investigations, in particular for ultrasound scanning as it wastes time and has false positives and negatives.

1. History: acutely swollen and painful testis, lower abdominal pain and sometimes vomiting (the abdominal pain occurs because the testis retains its embryological nerve supply which primarily is from the T10 sympathetic pathway). Recent mild trauma (that would not explain the pain), erection or intercourse. More frequent in teens, infants and also first year of life. The pain usually awakens the patient.

Past medical history: mild trauma to the testis, or previous episodes of testicular pain due to torsion and untwisting (de-torsion).

2. Physical examination (Fig. 4.): it's always difficult. High lying testis, extremely painful, swollen and thickened cord (difficult to feel). Normal contralateral testis.

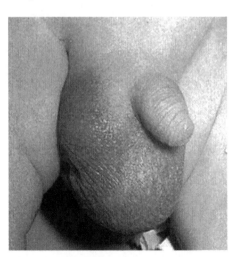

Fig. 4.1. Right testis torsion.

	Epididymo-orchitis	Testicular torsion
Age	Any, mostly adults	Children, young males, peak 13-15 years
Pain	Gradual, moderate to severe, tends to be confined to the epididymis	Acute, very severe (waking the patient up at night), localised in the testis
LUTS	+	-
Cremasteric reflex	-/+	-
Fever	+	-
Prehn's sign (Elevation of the affected testis relieves pain)	+	-
Skin change	Oedema and swelling of the scrotum	Rarely
Position of the testis	Normal but swollen	High and horizontal
Hx of trauma	Sometimes	More often

3. Investigations: none for diagnosis. Urine dip to rule out infection. There is no clinical value in preoperative Ultrasound scanning in suspected acute testicular torsion.

Differential diagnosis is with epididymo-orchitis (UTI chapter).

Treatment.
Testicular torsion is a urological surgical emergency. Scrotal exploration should be done as soon as possible (within 6 hours). Otherwise there will be irreversible testicular damage. This is a time sensitive diagnosis: establish as precisely as possible when the symptoms started. If more than 24 hours the risks of crash surgery (no fasting) may be higher than the possible benefits (testis will be necrotic). The amount of residual damage is proportional to the time between onset and correction.

The patient should be informed, and consented for orchiectomy (within the time constraints of an ischaemic emergency). During the operation: a high scrotal incision is recommended. The affected side presented under the skin incision, the tunica vaginalis is incised with scalpel and extended with scissors and the testis delivered. There is usually a small hydrocele. The torsion, if present, is immediately recognised and the cord is untwisted (first manoeuvre) and the testis placed between warm wet swabs. If viability is in doubt, wait a few minutes and re-examine. A gangrenous black testis that fails to recover its colour (after detorsion) is necrotic and must be removed and the cord transfixed; as autoantibodies may affect contralateral spermatogenesis (Fig. 4.2). If some blood supply and colour returns the testis may be viable and should be left. In this case the tunica vaginalis is resected or everted to prevent recurrence. Fixation with sutures between the albuginea and the dartos is not necessary. Through the same incision the opposite testis must be fixed at the same time and in the same way, as the predisposing anatomy tends to be bilateral.

Outcomes will depend on the state of tissue viability at the moment of de-torsion.

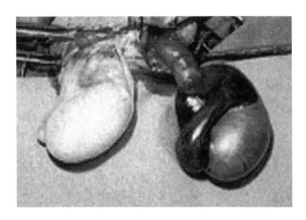

Fig. 4.2. Testicular exploration showing torsion of left testicle. It shows the difference between the viable and non-viable testis.

B. Torsion of the hydatid of Morgagni and the appendix epididymis.

Both can mimic testicular torsion, therefore, scrotal exploration is the safest management with excision of the epididymal appendix once torsion is ruled out.

Only ever not operate if you have very good reasons not to do so (time from onset, very clear clinical signs, surgical risk, unable to access adequate facilities). If available, ultrasound scanning can be reassuring.

At surgery, once torsion is ruled out, the affected appendix should be excised and the base diathermied or sutured. Fixation is not indicated but eversion of the tunica is.

Additional reading:

1. Acute scrotum in children. European Association of Urology. The Paediatric Urology Guidelines. http://uroweb.org/wp-content/uploads/23-Paediatric-Urology_LR_full.pdf. On 27/03/2016.
2. Testicular torsion: diagnosis, evaluation, and management. Sharp VJ, Kieran K, Arlen AM. Am Fam Physician. 2013 Dec 15; 88(12): 835-40.
3. Acute scrotal pain. Srinath H. Aust Fam Physician. 2013 Nov; 42(11): 790-2.
4. Acute scrotum. American Urological Association. https://www.auanet.org/education/acute-scrotum.cfm. On 21/03/2016.
5. Intermittent testicular pain: fix the testes. Kamaledeen S, Surana R. BJU Int. 2003 Mar; 91(4): 406-8.
6. Scrotal swellings. National Institute for Health and Care Excellence. https://www.evidence.nhs.uk/document?ci=http%3a%2f%2fcks.nice.org.uk%2fscrotal-swellings&returnUrl=Search%3fom%3d[{%22toi%22%3a[%22Guidance%22]}]%26q%3dScrotal%2bswellings&q=Scrotal+swellings. On 27/03/2016.
7. Testicular torsion. Cox AM, Patel H, Gelister J. Br J Hosp Med (Lond). 2012 Mar; 73(3): C34-6.
8. Testicular torsion. BMJ Best practice. http://bestpractice.bmj.com/best-practice/monograph/506.html. On 27/03/2016.

4.2. Paraphimosis.

Mr S Salloum and Mr G Shanmugham.

Definition.
Paraphimosis, also known as capistration, is the inability to bring the foreskin back to its original position after it is retracted behind the glans penis.

Aetiology.
It usually occurs with a tight preputial ring (phimosis) when it is retracted behind the glans. It also occurs commonly after procedures like catheterization when the foreskin is not repositioned forward after the procedure. It can also happen later in life when the ring tightens due to other pathology like balano-posthitis (e.g. in diabetics), balanitis xerotica obliterans (lichen sclerosus et atrophicus), etc. It is not uncommon for children to suffer from paraphimosis as the preputial orifice widens in the first years.

Diagnosis.
1. History: the prepuce forms a tight ring around the penis below the glans leading to oedema formation in the glans and below the coronal sulcus. Hence the common presentation is swelling and pain. Many young patients feel embarrassed to seek medical attention and will delay consultation and treatment and end up in severe discomfort and significant oedema.

2. Physical examination: oedema is noted at and below the glans penis and it is circumferential. The tight preputial ring is also noted. Penile oedema can at times be mistaken for paraphimosis in those who have been circumcised. In these patients oedema is noted below the glans but this oedema will be more dependent and predominantly ventral and if the patient is capable of giving a good history, he will recall having been circumcised in the past. (Fig. 4.3).

3. Investigations: the diagnosis is clinical, hence, none are required.

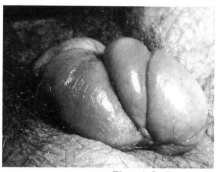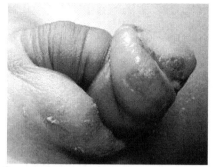

Fig. 4.3. Images of paraphimosis.

Treatment.

Involves bringing the foreskin back to normal position. For this to be achieved the oedema must be reduced and the prepuce pulled forward (distally). Since the patient will be in significant discomfort most patients need some form of anaesthesia either local or general. Children will need a general anaesthetic.

Medical.

Local anaesthesia can be given as a ring block around the base of the penis. Lidocaine or bupivacaine can be used but care must be taken to ensure that it does not contain adrenalin as penile ischaemia can result.

Circumferential penile block: this technique can be used for anaesthesia before attempting to manually reduce paraphimosis or any other painful penile procedures. Use a 27 gauge needle to circumferentially infiltrate local anaesthetic around the base of the penis, aspirate back to make sure that you are not in a blood vessel. Wait 5-10 min (go for a cuppa) and check the sensitivity and then you can start. Fig. 4.4.

Reduction of oedema: once anaesthesia has worked, the patient will be more co-operative for further manipulations. Reducing oedema can be achieved by manual compression after gauze soaked in iced cold saline solution is wrapped around the penis.

Reducing the prepuce: once the oedema is reduced, the prepuce can usually be brought forward to its normal position. This can be achieved by placing the index and middle fingers of both hands just

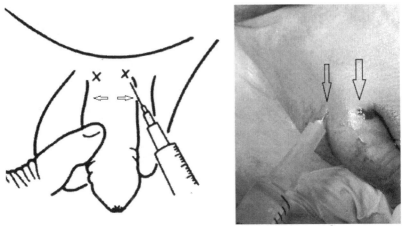

Fig. 4.4. Penile local anaesthetic ring block[3].

below the preputial ring on both sides of the shaft, and placing the thumbs on the glans. The four fingers push the preputial ring up while the thumbs push the glans down below the preputial ring, usually resulting in reduction of the paraphimosis. After reduction apply RICEN (Rest, Ice-packs, Compression, Elevation, and Non-steroidal analgesics). Fig. 4.5.

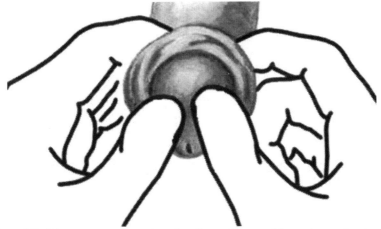

Fig. 4.5. Diagram: manual reduction of paraphimosis under local anaesthesia.

Surgical:
1. Dorsal slit: at times the above manoeuvres may not be successful. Then, the preputial ring will have to be cut to reduce the paraphimosis. Technique: the preputial ring will have to be slit laterally, or dorsally (para-medial), to avoid damaging the urethra

(ventrally) or the dorsal veins (medial, dorsally). The incision is made longitudinally and of sufficient length to reduce the paraphimosis (Fig. 4.6). Once it is reduced, the longitudinal incision is closed transversally so that the circumference of the preputial ring is increased; using absorbable suture material.

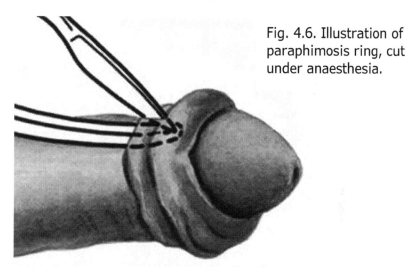

Fig. 4.6. Illustration of paraphimosis ring, cut under anaesthesia.

2. <u>Circumcision</u>: most patients will need a circumcision at a later date especially if the paraphimosis is recurrent or if there are any predisposing risk factors. Alternatively, a circumcision can be the initial treatment (instead of a slit cut) if reduction cannot be achieved. Fig. 4.7.

After surgical correction apply RICEN (Rest, Ice-packs, Compression, Elevation, and Non-steroidal analgesics).

Complications.
If a paraphimosis is unresolved for a long period, necrosis of the glans penis can result, with catastrophic consequences (partial amputation of the penis).

Outcomes.
Functional are generally good. Cosmetics may vary according to the technique used and will generally require further circumcision or preputioplasty.

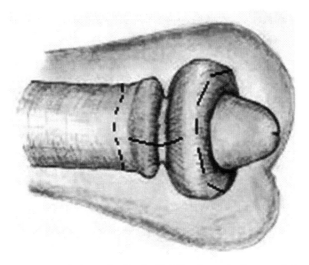

Fig. 4.7. Diagram of dorsal slit (solid line) and circumcision (dotted lines).

Additional reading:

1. Prepuce: phimosis, paraphimosis, and circumcision. Hayashi Y, Kojima Y, Mizuno K, Kohri K. ScientificWorldJournal. 2011 Feb 3; 11: 289-301.
2. Phimosis. European Association of Urology. The Paediatric Urology Guidelines. http://uroweb.org/wp-content/uploads/23-Paediatric-Urology_LR_full.pdf. On 27/03/2016.
3. Treatment options for paraphimosis. Little B, White M. Int J Clin Pract. 2005 May; 59(5): 591-3.
4. Paraphimosis. BMJ Best practice. http://bestpractice.bmj.com/best-practice/monograph/765.html. On 27/03/2016.
5. Penile emergencies. Dubin J, Davis JE. Emerg Med Clin North Am. 2011 Aug; 29(3): 485-99.

4.3. Priapism.

Mr S Salloum and Mr J Clavijo.

Definition.
Priapism is a relatively uncommon condition defined as a persistent pathological unwanted erection lasting more than 4 hours which is not associated with sexual desire or in the absence of sexual stimulation. Priapism is a urological emergency and requires a prompt and accurate evaluation and usually requires emergency treatment in order to offer the best chances to minimize the risk of future erectile dysfunction.

Aetiology.
1. Idiopathic.
2. Secondary:
   - Infection.
   - Trauma.
   - Neurogenic.
   - Coagulation disorders.
   - Medication.
   - Intracavernosal treatment of erectile dysfunction.
   - Bladder or prostate tumours.

Classification.
1. Ischaemic, veno-occlusive or low flow: it has the potential to cause erectile dysfunction damaging cavernous tissue consecutive to ischemic injury if it last more than 4 hours. Irreversible cellular damage with cavernosal fibrosis and impotence will also occur if treatment is delayed for more than 24 hours.
2. Non-ischaemic, arterial or high flow: it is a less common form of priapism and is often consequent to a traumatic lesion of the cavernosal artery or one of its branches within the corpus cavernosum. Cases with high-flow priapism due to needle laceration of the cavernosal artery during intracavernosal treatment are possible.
3. Recurrent or stuttering: is quite a rare type, characterized by alternation of erection and detumescence cycles. It is often seen in patients with sickle cell disease but could be also idiopathic.

Occasionally, this type could become ischaemic.

High Flow (arterial)	Low Flow (ischaemic)
Not painful	Painful
Well-oxygenated corpora cavernosa	Ischaemic corpora cavernosa
Adequate arterial flow	Inadequate arterial flow
Soft erections	Rigid erection
May be sexually active	Inactive sexually and without desire
Initiating event usually straddle injury	No history of trauma
May provide long history/situation,	Usually present to emergency room within hours
may be chronic in nature at presentation	High risk for erectile dysfunction (long-term)
Low risk for permanent injury/erectile dysfunction	Frequently associated with substance abuse or vasoactive penile injections
Rarely caused by medication	
Conservative management appropriate (initial) form of treatment	Conservative management inappropriate form of treatment
Consider elective embolization as treatment	Trial of adrenergic medication

Diagnosis.
Management of priapism depends on whether it is ischaemic or arterial. Resolution of priapism happens when the penis becomes flaccid and non-painful, spontaneously or after treatment. Recurrence of priapism happens when resolution lasts for at least 24 hours.

1. History: duration of priapism, pain, trauma. Also, patients with post-traumatic priapism typically have delayed onset (a few days), which is probably due to the segmental necrosis of the traumatized cavernosal artery over time leading to shunted blood flow.

Past medical history: haematological and thrombotic pathology such as sickle cell anaemia and other haemoglobinopathies and different

Main diagnostic criteria:

FINDINGS	ISCHAEMIC PRIAPISM	ARTERIAL PRIAPISM
Penile pain	Usually present	Rare
Abnormal cavernous blood gases	Venous	Arterial
Blood abnormalities and hematologic malignancy	Sometimes present	Very rare
Recent intracavernosal vasoactive drug injections	Sometimes present	Seldom present
Chronic, well tolerated tumescence without full rigidity	Rare	Usually present
Perineal trauma	Seldom present	Sometimes present

forms of leukaemia may lead to priapism. Malignancies can determine priapism by obstructing the venous outflow, the most common cancers involved being bladder transitional cell carcinoma, prostate adenocarcinoma, recto-sigmoid cancer and renal cell carcinoma. Neurological diseases such as spinal cord lesions or spinal stenosis may cause priapism. Drug history is extremely important. Currently, the use of intracavernosal injected agents for erectile dysfunction as Papaverin, Prostaglandin E1 (Alprostadil or PGE1), Phentolamine and other vasoactive drugs represents the most common cause of priapism. Rarely, PDE5 inhibitors (Avanafil, Sildenafil, Tadalafil, and Vardenafil) may produce it. Also drugs used to treat different diseases as antihypertensives, anticoagulants (heparin), antidepressants and antipsychotics may be associated with priapism.

2. Physical examination: evaluation of genitalia and perineum may reveal signs of a recent trauma which may suggest arterial priapism. In patients with priapism, the corpora cavernosa are rigid, while the corpus spongiosum and glans penis are not. Assessment of the corpus cavernosum, which is fully rigid in ischemic priapism and semi-rigid in arterial priapism, may help to determine the type of priapism. Tricorporal priapism (including corpus spongiosum) has been described due to sickle cell disease and primary and metastatic tumours of the penis. Abdominal and rectal examination can rule out the presence of other malignancies.

3. Investigations.
Blood tests: full blood count. Coagulation screen.
Corpora cavernosa blood gases:

Source	PO2(mmHg)	PCO2(mmHg)	pH
Ischemic priapism (cavernous blood)	<30	>60	<7.25
Arterial priapism blood	>90	<40	7.40
Normal cavernosal blood	40	50	7.35

Imaging.
- Penile duplex Doppler ultrasound: is useful in arterial priapism revealing the vascular abnormalities as fistulas or pseudo aneurisms. Cavernous blood flow is usually normal or somewhat increased. In ischemic priapism, ultrasonography will reveal absent or extremely low flow.
- Arteriography: could represent both a diagnostic and therapeutic method in patients with arterial priapism demonstrating the vascular defect and treating it by selective or super selective embolization.

Treatment.
Arterial priapism.
When history, examination and corpora cavernosa blood gases are suggestive of arterial priapism, an urgent arteriography is needed. If the diagnosis is confirmed, selective or super selective embolization is performed, at that moment or electively. Confirmed arterial priapism is not an emergency.

Ischaemic priapism.
A stepwise approach has been recommended starting with the least invasive treatment. Unlike arterial, ischaemic priapism is a real emergency.
1. Medical treatment.
- In the early stages of priapism, less than 4 hours since onset, ice packs, physical effort or cold showers may work (adrenergic

stimuli). If sickle cell crisis, resuscitate (pain control and IV fluids).
- Analgesia + Terbutaline 5-10 mg PO and wait 15 min.
- Give another dose and wait 15 min.
- Cavernosal blood aspiration: penile ring block local anaesthesia (as described in paraphimosis chapter). Then 20-40 ml of blood is aspirated with a 19 - 21 G butterfly needle and further aspirations should be done until bright red blood is obtained. Then irrigate the corpora cavernosa with normal saline for wash-out of hypoxic blood. Wait 5 to 10 min, if detumescence does not occur, intracavernosal injection of an α-adrenergic agent must be used (Phenylephrine). Before injection, Phenylephrine should be diluted with normal saline to a concentration of 100 to 500 µg/ml. Recommended protocol is to perform 1 ml injection every 3 to 5 minutes for approximately 1 hour until complete detumescence occurs (side effects can be flushing, headache, acute hypertension, reflex bradycardia, tachycardia, sweating and arrhythmia).

After detumescence apply RICEN (Rest, Ice-packs, Compression, Elevation, and Non-steroidal analgesics).

2. Surgical treatment.
Biopsy and corpora cavernosa-spongiosum shunts, as described below. Fig. 4.8 a and b, and 4.9.

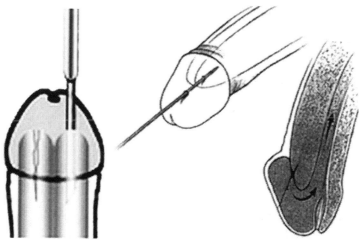

Fig. 4.8.a. Winters procedure.

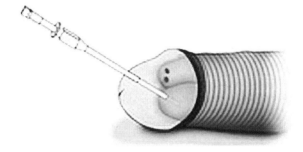

Fig. 4.8.b. Winters procedure: trans glans corpora cavernosa to spongiosum shunt performed with a wide bore needle.

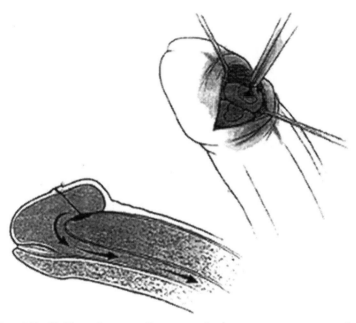

Fig. 4.9. Al Ghorab operation, surgical corpora cavernosa to spongiosum shunt. Usually done under general anaesthetic.

After surgical correction apply RICEN (Rest, Ice-packs, Compression, Elevation, and Non-steroidal analgesics).

If the above measures have not proven successful (unusual) then other surgical procedures must be considered including: corpora cavernosa-saphenous shunt, and insertion of a penile prosthesis (for prolonged priapism > 24 hours). Description of these last two is beyond the scope of this book.

Complications.
The main complication is corpora cavernosal fibrosis and subsequent end organ erectile failure. As with many emergencies, "time is tissue" holds true for priapism.

Outcomes.
Outcomes are inversely proportional to the duration of priapism. If unresolved in 24 hours, residual potency will be less than 20%.

Additional reading:

1. Acute management of priapism in men. Tay YK, Spernat D, Rzetelski-West K, Appu S, Love C. BJU Int. 2012 Apr; 109 Suppl 3: 15-21.
2. Standard operating procedures for priapism. Burnett AL, Sharlip ID. J Sex Med. 2013 Jan; 10(1): 180-94.
3. European Association of Urology guidelines on priapism. Salonia A, Eardley I, Giuliano F, Hatzichristou D, Moncada I, Vardi Y, Wespes E, Hatzimouratidis K; European Association of Urology. Eur Urol. 2014 Feb; 65(2): 480-9.
4. Unsatisfactory outcomes of prolonged ischemic priapism without early surgical shunts: our clinical experience and a review of the literature. Zheng DC, Yao HJ, Zhang K, Xu MX, Chen Q, Chen YB, Cai ZK, Lu MJ, Wang Z. Asian J Androl. 2013 Jan; 15(1): 75-8.
5. Guideline on the Management of Priapism. American Urological Association. http://www.auanet.org/common/pdf/education/clinical-guidance/Priapism.pdf. On 21/03/2016.
6. A pathophysiology-based approach to the management of early priapism. Kovac JR, Mak SK, Garcia MM, Lue TF. Asian J Androl. 2013 Jan; 15(1): 20-6.

CHAPTER 5. Trauma.

5.1. Renal and ureteral trauma.

Mr E M Paez and Mr P D Rimington.

A. Renal Trauma.

Definition.
Kidney injury produced by different mechanisms including blunt and penetrating trauma and iatrogenic interventions.

Aetiology.
Let's make this clear: you don't see this on a daily basis. It represents about 3% of all traumas. The vast majority (80-90%) are blunt. The mechanisms of blunt trauma could be via direct blow to the kidney, acceleration/deceleration injuries or both. Most common causes include RTA's, falls, contact sports and assault. Penetrating injuries include gunshot and stab wounds.

Classification.
AAST renal injury grading scale (Fig. 5.1).

Grade*   Description of injury.

1   • Contusion or non-expanding sub capsular haematoma
           • No laceration

2   • Non-expanding peri-renal haematoma
           • Cortical laceration < 1 cm deep without extravasation

3   • Cortical laceration > 1 cm without urinary extravasation

4   • Laceration: through corticomedullary junction into collecting system
                 or
           • Vascular: segmental renal artery or vein injury with contained haematoma, or partial vessel laceration, or vessel thrombosis

5   • Laceration: shattered kidney or
           • Vascular: renal pedicle avulsion
*Advance one grade for bilateral injuries up to grade III.

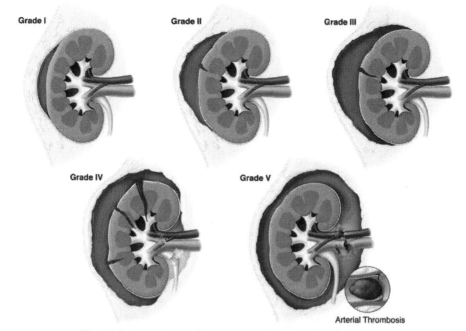

Fig. 5.1. AAST renal injury grading scale diagram.

Diagnosis.

High suspicion is the key to diagnosis. Undetected trauma can be fatal.

1. History: from patient, witnesses and emergency personnel including mechanism, nature and time of injury. Haematuria. Pain. In case of penetrating injuries try to establish type, size and direction of weapon, or type and calibre in gunshot wounds.

Past medical history and surgical history. Urological conditions. Drug history: anticoagulants, other medications and drugs.

2. Physical examination: blood pressure, pulse, pallor, shock (defined as systolic BP below 90 at any time during an adult patient's evaluation). Complete examination looking for penetrating wounds. Skin lesions including ecchymoses and abrasions (such as tyre treads). Fractures. Abdominal guarding or mass. Haematuria.

3. Investigations:

Blood: U&E, FBC.

Imaging: CT scan of abdomen with contrast and delayed phase films is the preferred imaging technique (Fig. 5.2). Indications for radiological evaluation:
a) Blunt abdominal trauma with visible haematuria or dipstick haematuria with systolic BP of less than 90 at any point.
b) Rapid deceleration injury and/or significant associated injuries.
c) Any degree of haematuria after penetrating abdominal or lower thoracic injury, or trajectory of weapon highly suggestive of renal involvement.

Look for: parenchymal lacerations and urinary extravasations, segmental parenchymal infarction, size and location of the surrounding retroperitoneal haematoma and associated abdominal injuries. Bone fractures are frequent, look for vertebral wing (transverse process) fractures.

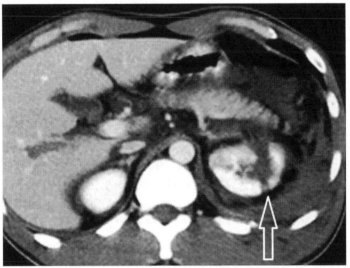

Fig. 5.2. CT shows grade 4 left renal lesion (arrow).
Others: dipstick. Haematuria is not the only decision factor.

Treatment.
ATLS or local trauma protocol assessment and management. Resuscitate. 80% of renal injuries are associated with liver trauma on the right side and with spleen trauma on the left.

Haemodynamic control and renal preservation are the aims of management. The tolerance for medical (non-operative) management has increased, even in the most seriously injured kidneys, to try to preserve residual renal function. Most renal contusions improve with bed rest, particularly if the lesion is of grade I-III. The closed retroperitoneal fossa facilitates tamponade of bleeding renal lacerations. If bleeding continues, in grade III-IV lesions, the use of selective embolization (Fig. 5.3) and percutaneous drainage of a significant or infected urinoma, if present, should be considered.

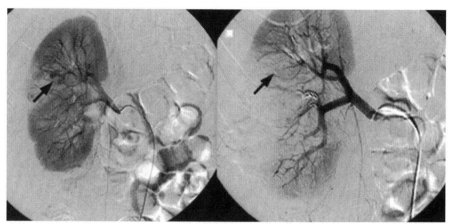

Fig. 5.3. Arteriogram with selective embolization of right renal artery branch (arrows).[4]

An exploratory laparotomy is needed **only** in patients with severe haemodynamic instability. In these, shock is usually due to associated injuries. Patients who require immediate surgical exploration should undergo one-shot, high-dose (2ml/kg of contrast) intravenous urography (IVU) on the surgical table, prior to any renal exploration. A single film is taken 10 minutes after the injection of contrast. The purpose is to determine the presence of 2 functioning renal units, the presence and extent of any urinary extravasation, and, in penetrating injuries, the likely course of the missile/blade. The finding of a retroperitoneal haematoma during laparotomy may indicate the presence of renal injury as does direct evidence of penetrating trauma. Always obtain early proximal vascular control. Repair of the affected kidney should be attempted whenever possible, and nephrectomy should be reserved for life threatening injuries when your attempts at renal preservation have failed.

Blunt Trauma. 5% requires urgent surgery.

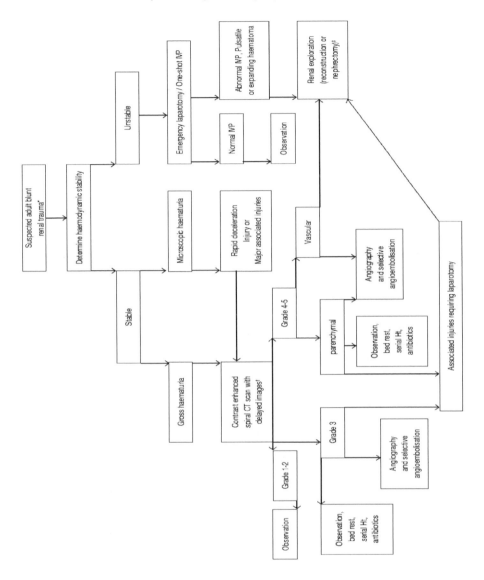

Penetrating Trauma. 50% requires urgent surgery.[5]

Always consider tetanus booster.

Complications.
Acute bleeding, infection, arterial-venous fistula, urinoma, delayed bleeding, urinary fistula, abscess, and later hypertension.

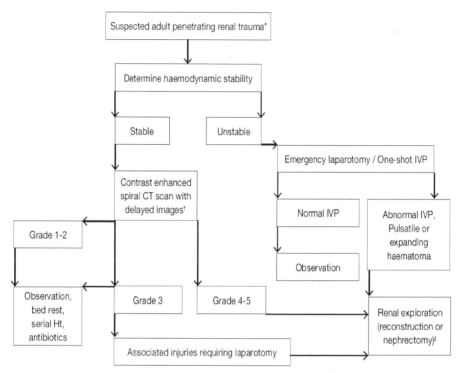

Penetrating trauma management.[6]

Outcomes.
This will depend on the extent of the lesion(s) and the success of the treatment. Follow up should include repeat imaging and reno-vascular hypertension screening, as well as renal function assessment.

B. Ureteral Trauma.

Definition.
Ureteral injury produced by different mechanisms including blunt and penetrating trauma and iatrogenic injury from surgical interventions.

Aetiology.
75% are iatrogenic, more commonly from urological, gynaecological, obstetric, colorectal and vascular procedures, 20% are caused by blunt trauma and 5% by penetrating. 75% involve distal ureter.

Mechanisms (Fig. 5.4): kinking, crushing, electro coagulation, perforation, ligation, total or partial section, excision, avulsion. Iatrogenic interventions include urological, gynaecological, obstetric, colorectal and vascular operations.

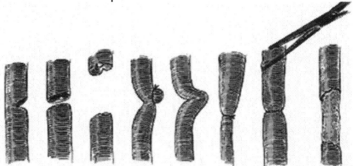

Fig. 5.4. Ureter lesions diagram.

Classification.
AAST Ureter injuries grading scale.

Grade. Description of injury.
1 Haematoma only
2 Laceration < 50% of circumference
3 Laceration > 50% of circumference
4 Complete tear < 2 cm of devascularisation
5 Complete tear > 2 cm of devascularisation

Diagnosis.
High suspicion is the key to diagnosis. 90% of injuries from external trauma are recognised in the first 24 hours, while this drops to 50% for surgical (iatrogenic) ones.

1. History: there are no typical symptoms related to ureteric trauma. Haematuria (50%- 75 %). Loin or abdominal pain or generalised distention can be present. High levels of suspicion in all cases of penetrating trauma and rapid deceleration.

Past medical history: recent operations. Drug history: anticoagulants.

2. Physical examination: findings are non-specific. Rule out associated lesions in abdomen and pelvis. Signs can include ileus, abdominal distention, frank peritonism and sepsis. In iatrogenic

cases, urine can leak from surgical wounds or drains.

3. Investigations.
Blood: creatinine from serum and surgical drain (if present). If urine leak, creatinine levels in drain fluid will be significantly higher than serum creatinine. FBC.

Imaging: CT with contrast and delayed films (Fig. 5.5) or IVU showing either obstruction or extravasation at the site of insult. Retrograde uretero-pyelogram if an intra-operative lesion is suspected.

Others: urinalysis (haematuria is not always present), urine culture.

Treatment.
Surgical exploration of the retroperitoneum with visualization of the ureter is the best method of diagnosing ureteral injury. Almost 90% of lesions can be detected this way.

Partial injuries Grade I-II can be treated with ureteric stent or placement of a nephrostomy to divert the urine. Stent for at least 3 weeks, imaging with contrast (IVU, CT urogram) and renogram 3-6 months later.

Intraoperative diagnosis: primary repair with a spatulated end to end, tension free anastomosis over a JJ stent is generally possible. Adjacent drain recommended. Rule out associated lesions in the abdomen and pelvis.

Postoperative diagnosis: if found within first week of insult, repair early and cover with antibiotics. If found later (delayed postoperative diagnosis) is best to leave a urine diversion via a nephrostomy or stent for 8-12 weeks with antibiotic coverage and repair later. Sub-acute tissue conditions (frailty and adhesions) make repair more difficult (facilitate ureter length loss).

Options for ureteric repair:
• Distal ureter: ureter re-implantation. Bladder mobilisation (psoas hitch) with or without a tubular flap (Boari flap) may be required for a tension free anastomosis over a JJ stent.

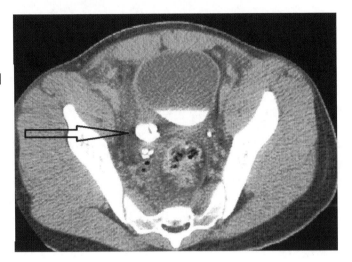

Fig. 5.5. Distal right ureter lesion in CT (arrow).

- Proximal ureter: spatulated end to end anastomosis or pelvic-ureteric anastomosis or uretero-calycostomy over a JJ sent. Again tension free.
- Extensive damage may require ileal ureter or auto transplant.

Complications.
Present in 25% of patients after repair. They include: extravasation, infection, urinoma, abscess, stricture, fistula and renal unit loss.

Outcomes.
Will depend on the nature and extent of the lesion and the response to the corrective procedure.

Additional reading:
1. Imaging of renal trauma: a comprehensive review. Kawashima A, Sandler CM, Corl FM, West OC, Tamm EP, Fishman EK, Goldman SM. Radiographics. 2001. May-Jun; 21(3): 557-74.
2. A review of ureteral injuries after external trauma. Pereira BM, Ogilvie MP, Gomez-Rodriguez JC, Ryan ML, Peña D, Marttos AC, Pizano LR, McKenney MG. Scand J Trauma Resusc Emerg Med. 2010 Feb 3;18:6.
3. Ureteral injuries: external and iatrogenic. Elliott SP, McAninch JW. Urol Clin North Am. 2006 Feb; 33(1): 55-66.
4. Injury Scoring Scales. The American Association for the Surgery of Trauma. http://www.aast.org/asset.axd?id=56ef079d-229c-45f2-9b18-c3825e450e65&t=633867256925730000. On 27/03/2016.
5. Urological Trauma. European Association of Urology Guidelines. http://uroweb.org/guideline/urological-trauma/. On 27/03/2016.
6. Selective management of Isolated and Non Isolated Grade IV Renal Injuries. Buckley, J; McAninch, J. JUrol, Issue 6, 2498-2502, Dec 2006.
7. Urotrauma. American Urological Association.

http://www.auanet.org/common/pdf/education/clinical-guidance/Urotrauma.pdf. On 21/03/2016.

8. The conservative management of renal trauma: a literature review and practical clinical guideline from Australia and New Zealand. McCombie SP, Thyer I, Corcoran NM, Rowling C, Dyer J, Le Roux A, Kuan M, Wallace DM, Hayne D. BJU Int. 2014 Nov; 114 Suppl 1: 13-21.

5.2. Pelvic trauma.

Mr S Salloum and Mr E M Paez.

A. Bladder Trauma.

Definition.
Injuries to the bladder resulting from several traumatic mechanisms.

Aetiology.
Frequency: 85% of patients with bladder injuries caused by blunt trauma have associated pelvic fractures, half of them are pubic rami ones.

A third of patients with pelvic fractures have bladder injuries and a third of those will be major ones. Most patients with pelvic fractures have multiple system injuries with a mortality of 1/3.

The distension of the bladder determines the injury it may have. A distended bladder can be ruptured by light pressure; however, an empty bladder is rarely injured. Rupture can be intra-peritoneal (with peritonitis) or sub-peritoneal.

Road traffic accidents (RTA) are one of the most common causes in urban areas. Other less common causes include industrial accidents, contact sports, gunshots and stab injuries. Iatrogenic lesions happen during obstetric, gynaecologic, urologic and colorectal surgery. Most can be diagnosed intra operatively and/or with cystoscopy and managed by adequate closure and drainage. In patients with bladder trauma due to a gunshot, the incidence of associated bowel injuries is as high as 83%. Colon injuries are reported in 33% of patients with stab wounds, and vascular injuries are as high as 82% in patients with a penetrating trauma (with a 63% mortality rate).

Classification.
Bladder injury scale.

Grade*   Description

I   Hematoma. Contusion, intramural hematoma, laceration partial thickness.

II   Laceration. Extra peritoneal bladder wall laceration <2 cm.

III   Laceration. Extra peritoneal (>2 cm) or intraperitoneal (<2 cm) bladder wall laceration.

IV   Laceration. Intraperitoneal bladder wall laceration >2 cm.

V   Laceration. Intraperitoneal or extra peritoneal bladder wall laceration extending into the bladder neck or ureteral orifice (trigone).

*Advance one grade for multiple injuries up to grade III.

Diagnosis.

1. History: triad of symptoms usually present includes:
    *   Haematuria. Note that up to 20% of bladder injuries can present without haematuria.
    *   Hypogastric pain/guarding.
    *   Dysuria, difficulty or even inability to void. The ability to urinate does not exclude bladder injury or perforation.

High level of suspicion in patients with complex pelvic or abdominal trauma. Try to establish mechanism of injury. Blunt trauma to the lower abdomen with a full bladder can cause intraperitoneal injuries without significant external signs.

Past medical history: urinary symptoms, previous surgery.

2. Physical examination: usually non-specific, lower abdominal pain and guarding can be present, bladder might not be palpable. Haematuria. Abdominal distention. Absent abdominal sounds. Ecchymoses and skin lesions.

3. Investigations:
Blood: FBC.

Imaging: CT retrograde cystogram (Fig. 5.6). It is diagnostic, and does not waste time. Contrast CT with delayed films with a full bladder will show contrast extravasation. Additional contrast can be added via urethral catheter. Under-filling (less than 250cc) of the bladder can give false negative results. The CT will also assess associated injuries in the abdomen and pelvis.

Good quality retrograde urethro-cystogram was the classic diagnostic method of bladder injuries, and it is still the modality of choice if associated urethral lesions are suspected.

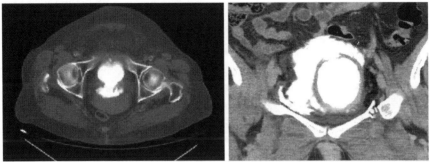

Fig. 5.6. CT images of bladder perforation.[7]

Others: urine dip for microscopic or visible haematuria.

Treatment.
Medical.
Resuscitate and stabilise. Trauma protocol. Rule out significant associated injuries.

Grade I-II injuries can be managed with urethral catheterisation, as long as there is no significant urine extravasation or signs of pelvic sepsis. A deferred retrograde urethrogram should be performed before catheter removal.

Surgical.
Grades III and IV need laparotomy with bladder closure and drainage. Grade V needs open reconstruction and drainage.

Always assess and manage associated injuries. Debride non-viable tissues. Make a watertight closure (check by filling the bladder through the urethral catheter). Keep catheter for at least a week before cystogram. Use adequate antibiotics, particularly in penetrating injuries and whilst having drainage tubes and catheter.

Complications.
Will be related to the lesion grade, but mainly to associated lesions, particularly vascular ones. They may also include urinary extravasation, fistulae, wound dehiscence, haematuria and pelvic infection.

Outcomes.

If managed promptly, bladder injuries per se are not life threatening. After recovery, detrusor and bladder neck function can be impaired and may need to be assessed, if the patient has persistent symptoms, via urodynamics.

B. Urethral Trauma.

Definition.

Injury to the urethra by several mechanisms. We describe here posterior urethral lesions. Anterior urethral lesions are described in external genital trauma.

Aetiology.

Posterior urethral trauma is usually associated with pelvic fractures. The incidence of urethral injury in pelvic fractures is 5-10% in men and 1-5% in women.

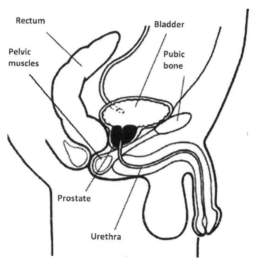

Fig. 5.7. Diagram of posterior urethra and pelvic muscles fascia.

During high impact injury, the membranous urethra is torn inferior to the pelvic floor muscles and fascia (bulbar-membranous junction). Fig. 5.7. Unstable pelvic and bilateral ischio-pubic rami fractures ("straddle"), and symphysis pubis and sacroiliac joint diastasis are highly likely to be associated to posterior urethral damage.

The posterior urethra can also be injured during endoscopic surgery (TURP, TURBT).

Classification.
Classification of blunt anterior and posterior urethral injuries:

Urethra injury scale

Grade*	Injury type	Description of injury
I	Contusion	Blood at urethral meatus; retrography normal
II	Stretch injury	Elongation of urethra without extravasation on urethrography
III	Partial disruption	Extravasation of urethrography contrast at injury site with visualization in the bladder
IV	Complete disruption	Extravasation of urethrography contrast at injury site without visualization in the bladder; <2cm of urethra seperation
V	Complete disruption	Complete transaction with >2 cm urethral separation, or extension into the prostate or vagina

Diagnosis.
1. History: patient presents with pelvic trauma and some of the following: red urethral bleeding, urinary retention, dysuria. With partial rupture voiding may be possible, but the urine will usually be bloody. The degree of haematuria is not always directly correlated to the extent of injury.

Past medical history: previous urethral pathology, STDs.

2. Physical examination: red urethral bleeding. Urinary retention (palpable bladder), dullness in lower abdomen could also represent a pelvic haematoma. High-riding prostate on rectal examination is a sign not always easy to identify. A large pelvic haematoma could be palpable as a boggy, indistinct mass. Assess associated injuries.

3. Investigations:
Blood: FBC.

Imaging:
1. Retrograde urethrogram (Fig. 5.8). Ideally performed with the

patient at 45 degrees and the penis stretched perpendicular to the femur. If due to the pelvis trauma this position is not possible, patient can be supine, with the penis stretched to one side.

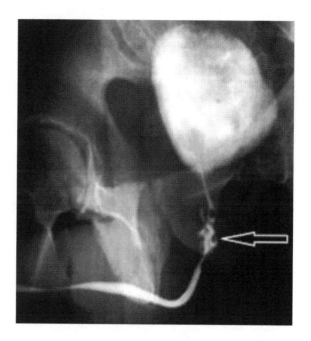

Fig. 5.8.
Urethrogram.
Posterior
urethral lesion
(arrow).

2. CT to assess associated lesions.

Others: urine dip for haematuria.

Treatment.
Medical.
Resuscitate and stabilise. Trauma protocol. Clinical management is according to the injury grade:
- Grade I no treatment required.
- Grades II and III can be managed conservatively with suprapubic cystostomy or urethral catheterization. With the latter consider the risk of converting a partial laceration to a total one, and introducing infection into a pelvic haematoma. Use of flexible cystoscopy and catheterisation over a guidewire in expert hands can be considered.

Surgical.
Treat electively whenever possible, draining the bladder initially via

supra-pubic catheter placed percutaneous or open. This has the lowest rate of ED. Urethral stricture is almost unavoidable, and this is repaired/treated electively.

Grades IV and V will require open or endoscopic treatment, primary or delayed. Grade V with extension into the prostate or vagina requires primary open repair.

Complications.
Complex and recurrent urethral strictures, sexual dysfunction, infertility and incontinence are typical late complications and will require elective tailored management.

Outcomes.
Will mainly depend on associated lesions on the acute stage and response to elective management of late complications.

Additional reading:
1. Current epidemiology of genitourinary trauma. McGeady JB, Breyer BN. Urol Clin North Am. 2013 Aug; 40(3): 323-34.
2. Injury Scoring Scales. The American Association for the Surgery of Trauma. http://www.aast.org/asset.axd?id=56ef079d-229c-45f2-9b18-c3825e450e65&t=633867256925730000. On 27/03/2016.
3. Urological Trauma. European Association of Urology Guidelines. http://uroweb.org/guideline/urological-trauma/. On 27/03/2016.
4. Urotrauma. American Urological Association. http://www.auanet.org/common/pdf/education/clinical-guidance/Urotrauma.pdf. On 21/03/2016.
5. Clinical review: initial management of blunt pelvic trauma patients with haemodynamic instability. Geeraerts T, Chhor V, Cheisson G, Martin L, Bessoud B, Ozanne A, Duranteau J. Crit Care. 2007; 11(1): 204.
6. Biomechanics of road traffic collision injuries: a clinician's perspective. Eid HO, Abu-Zidan FM. Singapore Med J. 2007 Jul; 48(7): 693-700.

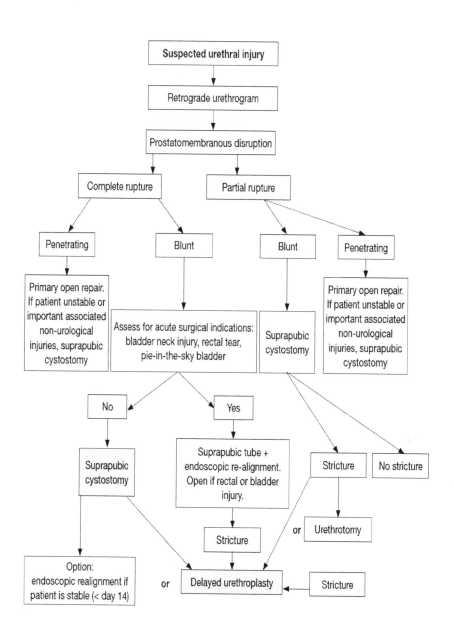

Posterior urethral injuries management.[8]

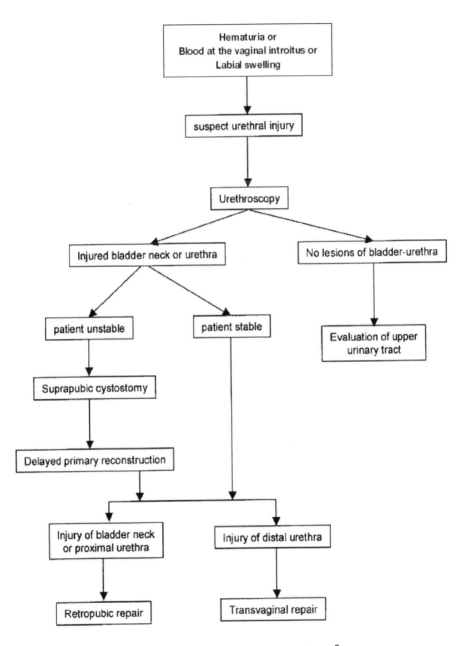

Female urethral trauma algorithm.[9]

5.3. External genital trauma.

Mr S Salloum, Mr P Verma and Mr J Clavijo.

Definition.
Penile or testicular injury produced by different mechanisms including blunt and penetrating trauma and iatrogenic interventions.

Aetiology.
It can be blunt, penetrating, avulsive (including mutilation), and also degloving in the scrotum or penis. Frequency: 40 to 50% of non-iatrogenic urology trauma. Mostly in young males. 80% blunt. Contact sports.

Classification.
A. Penile: penile fracture (during intercourse), zipper injuries (usually in children).
B. Urethral: anterior urethral injuries.
C. Scrotal: testicular and cord injuries.

A. <u>Penile Fracture and other Penile Trauma.</u>

The penis is rarely injured in the flaccid state. A violent thrust during erection against a rigid surface may lead to penile fracture. This condition is essentially a tear of the tunica of the corpus (or corpora) cavernosum.

Diagnosis.
1. History: a popping sound can be heard, early haematoma formation (aubergine sign), perineal butterfly ecchymoses, there may also be urethral bleeding. Pain of different degrees. Ask for nature and mechanism of trauma.

Past medical history: sexual practices, previous genital conditions. Drug history: anticoagulation, aspirin.

Penis injury scale

Grade*	Description of injury
I	Cutaneous laceration/contusion
II	Buck's fascia (cavemosum) laceration without tissue loss
III	Cutaneous avulsion
	Laceration through glans/meatus
	Cavemosal or urethral defect <2cm
IV	Partial penectomy
	Cavarnosal or urethral defect $\geq$ 2 cm
V	Total penectomy

*Advance one grade for multiple injuries up to grade III

2. Physical examination: typical extravasation of blood into the subcutaneous tissues of the penis (haematoma), pain on examination and angulation (Fig. 5.9). Perform EUA for full trauma assessment. Sometimes a triangle of normal skin (without hematoma) can be seen contralateral to the cavernosal tear.

3. Investigations:
Blood: FBC, coagulation screen.
Imaging: usually not necessary. Penile USS can show tunica tear. Retrograde urethrography should be performed if urethral injury is suspected. Cavernosogram is possible if in doubt.

Others: cystoscopy to assess urethra.

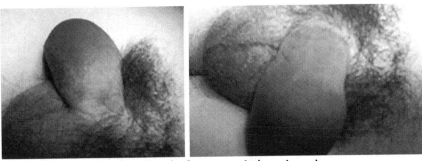

Fig. 5.9. Penile fracture. Aubergine sign.

Treatment.
Medical.
Stabilization of the trauma patient takes priority and may delay the care of penile injuries. Adequate dressings, appropriate wound

cultures, and tetanus prophylaxis are indicated in the interim. In animal bites consider rabies treatment. In human bites the risk of viral transmission is low. Still consider hepatitis B treatment and HIV post exposure prophylaxis.

Subcutaneous haematoma, without rupture of the cavernosal tunica albuginea (no immediate detumescence of the erect penis) and integrity of the skin, can be managed with RICEN (Rest, Ice-packs, Compression, Elevation, and Non-steroidal analgesics).

Zipper injuries can be dealt with by cutting the zipper, always under adequate anaesthesia.

Surgical.
Aim to prevent erectile dysfunction, maintain penile length, and allow normal (standing) voiding.

Penile fracture: immediate surgical intervention with closure of the tunica albuginea (Fig. 5.10).

Penetrating penile trauma: surgical exploration and conservative debridement of necrotic tissue is recommended with primary closure in most cases.

In amputation, consider re-implantation (if feasible) by an expert team. Clean organ with saline, wrap in wet swab and place in sterile plastic bag. Then place this bag inside another one containing ice or preferably frozen saline. This prolongs tissue survival.

Always use full antibiotic coverage. Treat associated lesions in abdomen, pelvis and perineum. In the postoperative period, benzodiazepines, Stilboestrol, LHRH blockers or Ketoconazole can be used to reduce the incidence of erections during recovery.

Complications.
Haematoma, infection, urethral fistula, sexual dysfunction.

Outcomes.
Cosmetics and cavernosal erectile capacity will depend on the extension of lesions and response to repair.

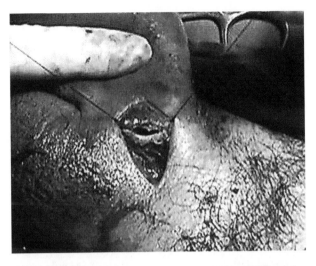

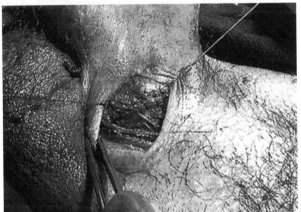

Fig. 5.10. Suture repair of corpus cavernosum tear.

B. Anterior Urethral Injuries.

Aetiology: blunt trauma to the perineum (straddle injuries), many have a delayed manifestation, as a urethral stricture. External penetrating trauma to the urethra is rare, but iatrogenic injuries are common. Most are related to difficult urethral catheterizations and transurethral procedures.

Diagnosis.
1. History: there may be urethral bleeding. Pain of different degrees. Difficulty in urination. Haematoma. Check nature and mechanism

of trauma. Are there penile or scrotal lesions?
Past medical history: previous urological conditions.

Urethra injury scale

Grade*	Injury type	Description of injury
I	Contusion	Blood at urethral meatus; retrography normal
II	Stretch injury	Elongation of urethra without extravasation on urethrography
III	Partial disruption	Extravasation of urethrography contrast at injury site with visualization in the bladder
IV	Complete disruption	Extravasation of urethrography contrast at injury site without visualization in the bladder; <2cm of urethra seperation
V	Complete disruption	Complete transaction with ≥2 cm urethral separation, or extension into the prostate or vagina

*Advance one grade for bilateral injuries up to grade III

American Association for Surgery of Trauma (AAST) classification.

2. Physical examination: perform EUA for full trauma assessment.

3. Investigations:
Blood: FBC, coagulation screen.

Imaging: retrograde urethrography should be performed. Look for location and extent of urethral defect(s) and urinoma.

Others: cystoscopy to assess urethra.

Treatment.
Medical.
Stabilization of the trauma patient takes priority and may delay the care of anterior urethral injuries.

Surgical.
Partial closed injuries can be managed with a SPC. The same treatment applies to female urethral injuries that are usually associated with vaginal lesions.

Penetrating anterior urethral injuries should be explored. Defects longer than 1.5 cm in the penile urethra should be repaired electively with reconstruction; otherwise debride and repair over a catheter as a primary measure. Always use full antibiotic coverage. Treat associated lesions in abdomen, pelvis and perineum.

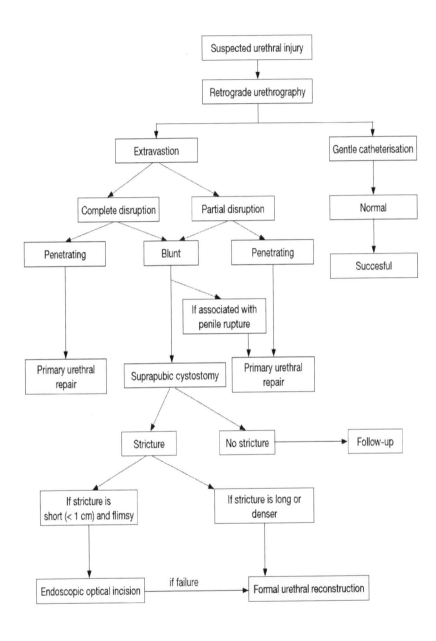

Management of anterior urethral injuries in men.[10]

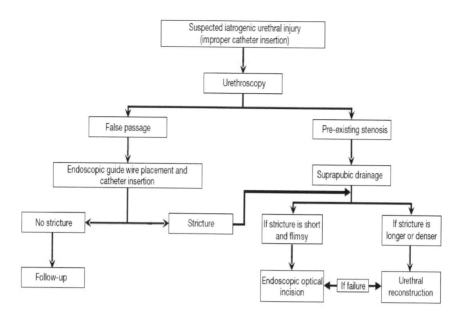

Iatrogenic urethral trauma algorithm.[11]

Complications.
Stricture, haematoma, infection, urethral fistula, sexual dysfunction.

Outcomes.
Will depend on the extension of lesions and response to repair. Elective management of resulting strictures tends to have a good prognosis.

C. Scrotal Trauma.

Frequency: testicular rupture in 50% of blunt scrotal trauma. Contact sports. Assault. Blunt injuries include dislocation (uncommon).

Diagnosis.
1. History: pain. Haematoma. Look for associated lesions.
Past medical history: previous genital conditions or operations. Drug history: anticoagulation.

2. Physical examination: as in the penis, there is subcutaneous haematoma, pain on examination and skin lesions in penetrating

injuries. Perform EUA for full trauma assessment.

3. Investigations:
Blood: FBC, coagulation screen.

Testis injury scale

Grade*	Description of injury
I	Contusion/hematoma
II	Subclinical laceration of tunica albuginea
III	Laceration of tunica albuginea with <50% parenchymal loss
IV	Major laceration of tunica albuginea with $\geq$50% parenchymal loss
V	Total testicular destruction or avulsion

*Advance one grade for bilateral lesions up to grade V

American Association for Surgery of Trauma (AAST) classification.

Imaging: scrotal USS. Retrograde urethrography, if urethral injury is suspected.

Others: EUA, including cystoscopy.

Treatment.
Medical.
Stabilization of the trauma patient often delays care of scrotal trauma. Dressings, wound cultures, and tetanus prophylaxis are indicated prior to definitive therapy. As above, in animal bites consider rabies treatment; consider hepatitis B treatment and HIV post exposure prophylaxis in human bites.

Minimal trauma with or without haematoma, and without testis rupture and integrity of the skin, can be managed, as in penile trauma, with RICEN (Rest, Ice-packs, Compression, Elevation, and Non-steroidal analgesics).

Surgical.
Indications for scrotal exploration (Fig. 5.11): uncertainty in diagnosis, suspicion of testicular rupture, disruption of the tunica albuginea, absence of blood flow on USS, haematoceles of over 3-5 cm, penetrating trauma.

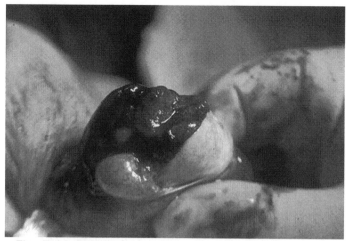

Fig. 5.11. Testicular rupture. Tunica albuginea tear.

In cases of penetrating trauma explore and perform antisepsis and debridement. When there is testicular rupture, do a testicular repair. Always use full antibiotic coverage. Treat associated lesions as per trauma protocol. In amputation, consider microsurgical re-implantation (if feasible) by an expert team. As for penile, clean organ with saline, wrap in wet swab and place in sterile plastic bag. Then place this bag inside another one containing ice or preferably frozen saline. This prolongs tissue survival.

Complications.
Infection, haematoma, testicular atrophy with or without impaired fertility, chronic orchidalgia.

Outcomes.
Better chance of testis salvage with an early intervention.

Additional reading:
1. Urotrauma. American Urological Association.
    http://www.auanet.org/common/pdf/education/clinical-guidance/Urotrauma.pdf. On 21/03/2016.
2. Injury Scoring Scales. The American Association for the Surgery of Trauma.
    http://www.aast.org/asset.axd?id=56ef079d-229c-45f2-9b18-c3825e450e65&t=633867256925730000. On 27/03/2016.
3. Urological Trauma. European Association of Urology Guidelines.
    http://uroweb.org/guideline/urological-trauma/. On 27/03/2016.
4. Traumatic penile injury: from circumcision injury to penile amputation. Kim JH, Park JY, Song YS. Biomed Res Int. 2014; 2014: 375285.
5. Doppler applications in testicular and scrotal disease. Dudea SM, Ciurea A, Chiorean

A, Botar-Jid C. Med Ultrason. 2010 Mar; 12(1): 43-51.

6. Male genital injury: diagnostics and treatment. van der Horst C, Martinez Portillo FJ, Seif C, Groth W, Jünemann KP. BJU Int. 2004 May; 93(7): 927-30.

CHAPTER 6. Surgical Complications in Urology.

6.1. Intra-operative complications.

Their prevention and clinical management.

Mr J Clavijo.

"If you don't know where you're going, you might wind up somewhere else." Yogi Berra.

Definition.
Intraoperative complications are adverse events that happen during a surgical or endoscopic procedure. They can occur even when due diligence is applied in following the adequate technical steps of the planned operation or procedure (even if everyone does everything right).

Aetiology.
Several factors predispose the occurrence of an adverse event (or omission). Most are human related, mainly to surgical team members. They include: distractions, inappropriate environment, difficult patient (case) or pathology, inadequate technique, standards, safety culture, staffing, skill mix, workload, equipment availability and maintenance, support, induction and mentoring, communication, and members' health (acute or chronic conditions).

Classification.
There have been attempts at classifying according to whether the event resulted in harm or not, particularly when looking at postoperative outcomes. Satava proposed a simple and useful classification to grade surgical errors during an operation:
Grade I: an error without consequence or a near miss.
Grade II: an error with immediate identification and correction, or recovery.
Grade III: an error that is unrecognized that leads to a significant consequence or complication.

Diagnosis.
The diagnosis will depend on the findings on each procedure. Awareness of the flow of the procedure and possible complications makes diagnosis easier, and earlier, at a stage where corrections are

also easier to implement.

Treatment.
The best way to manage a complication is to avoid it. Having said so, if you never had one, you have not been in the profession long enough (or treated enough cases).

When a complication is recognized the efforts have to be directed towards stopping it or preventing its progression. Simultaneously, actions have to be taken to secure patient's and organs' integrity and to eliminate any predisposing factors that led to the complication, as explained in aetiology.

1. Uncontrolled bleeding.

All surgical procedures and particularly excisional ones may involve control and section of vascular structures. When there is an unusual anatomical variant or when exposure is difficult, an artery, vein or highly vascular organ may be injured and bleed. Ideally, this should be foreseen and if possible, avoided. When a serious bleeding occurs, all members of the team should be informed (loud and clear). The scrub nurse should order all the necessary extra instruments and the anaesthetist reperfuse the patient. Request specific instruments for vascular repair, including: fine-tipped needle holder to take small needles, atraumatic vascular clamps designed to occlude blood vessels and suitable sutures. If an additional assistant is needed, he/she should be summoned in. Make sure everyone in theatre is fit for purpose and they are 100% focused on their task. Communication should be prompt, clear, brief and strictly to the point. Unlike in elective vascular surgery, a vascular complication during urological surgery needs good vascular exposure in an unplanned situation. Pressure with a large swab on the bleeding area will temporarily allow for redirecting the team's efforts to obtain haemostasis. Even the Aorta can be compressed close. Adequate exposure must be obtained to understand the type of lesion that needs repair. A poorly exposed operative field can lead to further injury. Once good exposure is achieved, attention should be focused to secure a proximal and distal vascular control. The swab should be slowly removed and the bleeding structure controlled and securely ligated or repaired. In all vascular repairs preserve a good vascular calibre to maintain adequate flow (transverse sutures).

If doing a laparoscopic procedure, increase the pressure to 20 mm Hg until haemostasis is achieved and add as many ports (and assistants) as necessary. Remember to lower the pressure after the repair. Minor and moderate laparoscopic complications can sometimes be controlled with laparoscopy by a **very experienced** surgeon. In all other scenarios the best and safer approach is to convert the operation to open to resolve the complication.

Renal artery. Even well tied knots can slip. Do not rely on them. A transfixion suture and double ligation (both sides) will never slip. If using clips: metallic ones are the least reliable. Always use 3 to the side of the patient and one on the specimen. The same applies to polymer ones. Use the correct size, and position and lock well. The correct functional length of a clip has to be slightly longer than half the circumference of the vessel to be controlled, not its diameter (which is what is seen). The correct position is perpendicular to the vessel. The close proximity of the superior mesenteric artery and left renal vein is well known and clearly plays a role in the confusion between the superior mesenteric artery and the left kidney artery.

IVC or renal veins. Again, do not rely on simple knots. Always have a good distance to cut through sutures. The right renal vein is short, so dissect very accurately. If in doubt, get a Satinsky clamp at the IVC. The left renal vein has several branches (gonadal, lumbar, adrenal) and they all have to be addressed. Renal veins, like arteries, can be multiple, so look for them. An astute Radiologist may warn you in advance. A good team makes life easier. If the IVC is injured, after the initial compression, a Satinsky clamp will allow repair with 4-0 Polypropylene sutures. If the defect is extensive, proximal and distal transverse clamping may be needed to allow for repair with or without a graft. Always seek the opinion and help of a vascular surgeon if at all possible. It is the right policy, and leads to better results for everyone. The use of stapling devices has become common. They can fail as much as polymer clips, and require as much dissection. If a device fails, don't waste time and secure a Satinsky in the IVC.

Santorini plexus. Sometimes more stitches means more bleeding. Compression and pinpoint ("selective") control with fine sutures is probably the better option.

Partial nephrectomy. Again, superb exposure is of the essence. The artery or arteries must be completely occluded in a non-traumatic way. Use cold ischaemia; it was invented for a reason. Vein control is frequently necessary on the right. With adequate vascular control the kidney will bleed only the blood it has inside it (and it is a sponge). After the resection and suturing, use oxidized cellulose (Surgicel®) bolsters and/or thrombin plus cross-linked gelatine (Floseal®), or similar products. Be safe, always. It is better than being sorry occasionally.

PCNL. An immediate or delayed bleeding can be an arterio-venous fistula. It will require an arteriogram and selective embolization.

2. Anaesthetics.

They include: MI, DVT/PE. Use DVT prophylaxis with TED stockings, pneumatic calf pumps (Flowtron®), peroneal nerve stimulation (Geko® device) and/or anticoagulants (Clexane®). Cross-consult early. Compartment syndrome, due to prolonged limb compression, is usually avoided by padding and the use of pneumatic pumps. If suspected, contact the Orthopaedic team on call as it may require fasciotomy.

During laparoscopic operations pneumothorax, respiratory acidosis and air embolism can occur.

3. TURP Syndrome (iatrogenic dilution hyponatremia).

During TUR (Fig. 6.1), the irrigation fluid is usually Glycine solution (Sorbitol and water are now rarely used). If absorbed in large amounts due to a prolonged procedure or opening of veins, it can lead to clinical symptoms of dilution hyponatremia. 1.5% Glycine is also hypotonic (200 mOsmol/l). In a TURP, there is approximately 20 ml/min absorption. Therefore, in a long, 60 minute resection, 1.2 L of Glycine solution is absorbed. This much can be coped with in a patient without comorbidities.

Symptoms include nausea, vomiting, headache and malaise, which are easily detectable if the patient has a regional anaesthesia. For this reason, regionals are the urologists' preferred anaesthesia for TURP. General anaesthesia masks these initial symptoms leading to a late diagnosis.

Dilution hyponatremia is the accepted cause of the syndrome and the symptoms do not appear until the concentration of sodium in serum falls below 125 mEq / L. Hypertension and confusion are predominant, then hypotension and bradycardia secondary to hyponatremia.

If the venous sinuses are open or capsular perforation occurs during resection, a loop diuretic should be given (Furosemide 40-120 mg). Note that the hyperosmolar nature of Mannitol can cause rapid expansion of intravascular volume. The extravascular fluid is then absorbed quicker increasing hyponatremia.

If hyponatremia is severe, there can be confusion, convulsions, stupor and coma, pulmonary oedema and cardiac failure secondary to fluid overload. Glycine related symptoms are flashing lights, prickling sensations and facial redness. If the patient is under general anaesthetic, hypertension from fluid overload may be the only sign. Due to the low osmolality, there can be haemolysis. This in turn produces jaundice, haemoglobinuria, acute renal failure, and anaemia. Once the diagnosis is made, the patient will need ultrafiltration, hence a timely consultation with the nephrologist / intensivist, is of order. The Urologist should lead the treatment team, as other specialists rarely see this complication. Management: Furosemide +/- ITU.

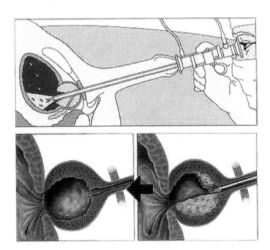

Fig. 6.1. TURP diagram.

With the use of bipolar resectoscopes, normal saline can be used instead of non-ionic and hypotonic solutions. This prevents both hyponatremia and hypo-osmolar haemolysis. **It does not reduce the**

amount of fluid absorbed during the TUR, so there is still the risk of intravascular volume overload in lengthy resections. The posterior part of the bladder neck is a common place of perforation and fluid absorption, when the circular fibres are seen, the resection should be discontinued. The adenoma is thinner in the anterior sector and perforation should be avoided at this level, where there are multiple venous sinuses, early entry into these can lead to a TUR syndrome.

A suprapubic (Reuter) trocar in the bladder can massively reduce the risk of absorption (Venturi effect). However, if the adenoma is too big (over 80 ml), the patient is better served by an alternative, suitable technique rather than a TURP.

4. Bladder perforation during TUR.

How far a resection of a bladder tumour should go is a matter of debate. Some surgeons "comb" the bladder and not unexpectedly, rarely have muscle in the histology report. A useless resection. On the other extreme if the histology reads: peri-vesical fat not involved, though quite reassuring, it may mean a perforation has occurred. Most sub-peritoneal perforations are easily dealt with by leaving an indwelling catheter for 5 to 10 days and avoiding postoperative intra-vesical chemotherapy. Intraperitoneal perforation is avoided by stopping the resection at the detrusor level in the areas in contact with peritoneum (anterior and superior walls). If an intra-peritoneal perforation happens and is immediately recognised, the procedure is stopped and it can be managed as a sub-peritoneal one but under strict vigilance to rule out peritonitis (Fig. 6.2). If it is delayed, big, or there are any suspicious signs of peritonitis, a laparotomy, peritoneal lavage and bladder closure is necessary.

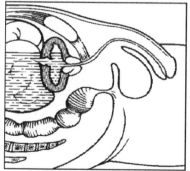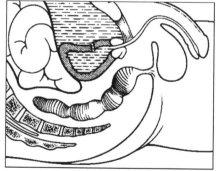

Fig. 6.2. Intra and sub-peritoneal bladder perforations.[12]

5. Spleen, liver and bowel lesions.

Intra-abdominal structures can be damaged during urological procedures. The descriptions of all of them as well as the remedial procedures are beyond the scope of this book. To avoid them, get good exposure, retract organs carefully, avoid using energy near the bowel, dissect (do not tear), protect abdominal organs and treat them as you would like the General Surgeons and Gynaecologists to treat the urinary tract. In laparoscopic procedures always keep instruments within the field of view, particularly scissors, loaded needle-holders and ultrasonic shears, they cause havoc when unattended.

6. Sepsis.

It is usually a postoperative complication. Work in and leave a clean operative field, leave drains and use antibiotic prophylaxis. Remove clots from the operative field before closure. Do not leave de-vascularized tissues behind. (See Chapter 1.6).

7. Ureteral avulsion.

It is a typical complication of ureteroscopy (Fig. 6.3). It usually happens when scoping in a non-stented and non-dilated ureter. If there is resistance to the advance of the scope, stop, insert a JJ stent and re-book. When it happens, the avulsion is usually near the vesico-ureteric junction, so the safest management is to do a ureteral re-implantation over a stent.

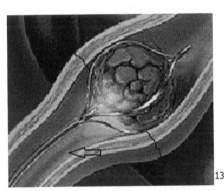

Fig. 6.3. Ureter avulsion during basket extraction. Direction of force (arrow).

8. Bladder and ureter injuries during gynaecologic operations.

Caesarean sections and hysterectomies account for the major part of bladder and ureteric injuries. When recognised intra-operatively, a careful dissection of the structures is necessary, multi-layer no-tension closure, bilateral JJ stenting and a urethral catheter and/or cystostomy would normally allow adequate healing after repair. If the distal ureter is considerably damaged, a ureteral re-implantation is the safer approach.

You are there to fix a problem (to a patient). Incident analysis and education do not have a place during intra-operative complication repair.

9. False passage.
This happens when the urethra is torn in an attempt at catheterisation or dilatation (Fig. 6.4). Blood is seen at the urethral meatus. Expert hands can attempt a trial to advance a thin catheter with variable success. The safe solution is the placement of a supra-pubic catheter either percutaneous or open (cystostomy).

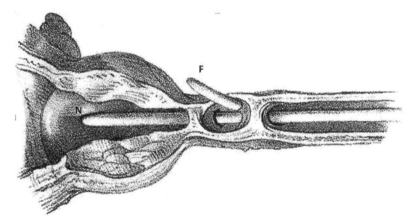

Fig. 6.4. Normal (N) and false (F) passage of a catheter with urethral damage.

10. Broken instruments and needles.
Even when carefully checked before use, some instruments may reach the end of their lifetime during an operation. Both disposable and reusable ones do break and fragments may disappear in the surgical field. The best option is a thoughtful search. If the fragment is metallic or a needle is lost, an x-ray film may aid in localisation (Fig. 6.5). If not found, everything must be explained in the surgical notes and the patient informed when recovered. We intentionally leave clips and other surgical devices (with specific purposes), during

an operation, and usually nothing happens afterwards. So one may presume that the same may occur with a lost fragment or needle.

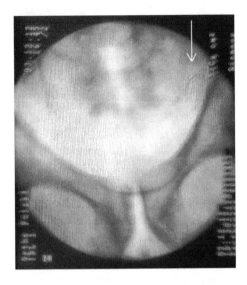

Fig. 6.5. Radioscopy showing needle (white arrow).

11. Complications during laparoscopic or lumboscopic (retroperitoneal) Urology.

Complications associated with these procedures are 4.4%, with a reoperation rate of 0.8% and a mortality rate of 0.08%. The complication rate increases in parallel with the difficulty of the procedure, but is inversely proportional to the experience of the surgeon.

Prevention.

All members of the team must be in a briefing planning session before the operation and at debriefing at the end of the procedure.

Know surgical anatomy well. Step progression with excellent exposure and haemostasis is the basis of surgical success. Only take strictly necessary risks, unfortunately this only comes with a high mileage of experience.

WHO Surgical Checklist.

This simple checklist is a safety instrument to run before the operation (Fig. 6.6). It is usually ticked by one of the circulating nurses and all the team members contribute to it. Priceless. It was designed as a starting point, so you can (and should) modify it to the needs of your team/specialty.

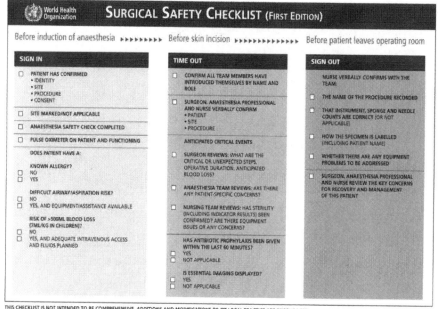

Fig. 6.6. WHO Surgical Checklist.

Additional reading:

1. Decision making in urological surgery. Abboudi H, Ahmed K, Normahani P, Abboudi M, Kirby R, Challacombe B, Khan MS, Dasgupta P. Int Urol Nephrol. 2012 Jun; 44(3): 701-10.

2. The use of haemostatic agents and sealants in urology. Hong YM, Loughlin KR. J Urol. 2006 Dec; 176(6 Pt 1): 2367-74.

3. Ureteric injury: a challenging condition to diagnose and manage. Abboudi H, Ahmed K, Royle J, Khan MS, Dasgupta P, N'Dow J. Nat Rev Urol. 2013. Feb; 10(2): 108-15.

4. Identification and reduction of surgical error using simulation. Satava RM. Minimally Invasive Therapy and Allied Technologies. 2005. 14; 4-5: 257–261.

5. Complications of laparoscopic procedures in urology: experience with 2,407 procedures at 4 German centers. Fahlenkamp D, Rassweiler J, Fornara P, Frede T, Loening SA. J Urol. 1999 Sep; 162(3 Pt 1): 765-70.

6.2. Post-operative complications.

Their prevention and clinical management.

Dr R Molina, Mr S Salloum and Mr J Clavijo.

"The incidence of postoperative complications is still the most frequently used surrogate marker of quality in surgery."
Pierre-Alain Clavien.

Definition.
Post-operative complications are adverse events that happen after a surgical or endoscopic procedure. They are deviations from the normal postoperative course. They can occur even when due diligence is applied in following the adequate technical steps of the planned operation or procedure (even if everyone does everything right).

Aetiology.
Like in intra-operative complications, this is multifactorial including acts and omissions. Most are human related. They include: distractions, inappropriate environment, difficult patient or pathology, inadequate standards and safety culture, staffing, skill mix, workload, equipment maintenance, and communication. Anaesthetic complications are many and lay beyond the scope of this book. They include: pneumonia, atelectasis, and acute cardiac ischaemia.

Classification.
The Clavien-Dindo Classification of Surgical Complications is the preferred one for postoperative events.
Grade I: any deviation from the normal postoperative course without the need for pharmacological treatment or surgical, endoscopic and radiological interventions. Allowed therapeutic regimens are: drugs as antiemetics, antipyretics, analgesics, diuretics and electrolytes and physiotherapy. This grade also includes wound infections opened at the bedside.
Grade II: requiring pharmacological treatment with drugs other than such allowed for grade I complications. Blood transfusions and total parenteral nutrition are also included.

Grade III: requiring surgical, endoscopic or radiological intervention.
Grade IV: life-threatening complication (including CNS complications) requiring ITU management.
Grade V: death of a patient.

1. Generic post-operative complications.

A. Infection.

Diagnosis.
History: temperature and or purulent drain/discharge after a procedure. It can also present with systemic symptoms. More frequent in contaminated/emergency operations. Past medical history: immune suppression.

Physical examination: look for abscesses, discharge, and peritonitis. Temperature curve, which is invaluable.

Investigations: blood culture, FBC. Imaging: usually CT if no focus is found clinically.

Treatment.
Medical: broad spectrum antibiotics covering presumed germs until microbiology information becomes available (urine, blood and drain cultures).

Surgical: drain any collections, "Ubi pus, ibi evacua" is still perfectly valid. Do it promptly.

Antibiotic prophylaxis in urological surgery.
Always obtain a Urine Dip-Test or Mid-Stream Urine Test (Dip/MSU) prior to any urological surgery. Check your local protocol, which depends on your local microbiological flora and the result of the MSUs and C&Ss. Patients with heart valve disease are likely to require: 1g Amoxicillin + 3 mg/kg of Gentamycin I/V at the induction of anaesthesia. If in doubt, follow Guidelines.

B. DVT + PE.

Diagnosis.
History: DVT symptoms: low grade fever, calf swelling and tenderness or pain. PE symptoms: dyspnoea, pleuritic chest pain and

haemoptysis. More prevalent in pelvic operations, particularly if long. Past medical history: previous DVT/PE, coagulopathies.

Physical examination: legs (pain, swelling, inflammation, circumference), tachycardia, tachypnea, high JVP, hypotension, pleural rub and pleural effusion.

Investigations: blood: D-dimers, ABG (low PO2, low PCO2).
Imaging: Doppler USS legs (urgent). CXR: normal or linear atelectasis, dilated pulmonary artery, reduced perfusion of affected segment, pleural effusion. CT pulmonary angiogram: it has better specificity and sensitivity than V/Q radioisotope scan. A negative CT pulmonary angiogram (CTPA) rules out a PE with similar accuracy to a normal isotope lung scan or a negative pulmonary angiogram.
ECG: This shows tachycardia, RBBB (inverted T in V1-V4) S1,Q3,T3.

Treatment.
Below-knee DVT: above-knee thromboembolic stockings (AK-TEDs), if no peripheral arterial disease (enquire for claudication and check pulses) + non-fractioned heparin 5000 IU S/C BID.
Above-knee DVT: start a low molecular weight heparin (i.e. Enoxaparin 1.5 mg/kg - 150 units/kg OD) until adequate oral anticoagulation is established (like Warfarin 10 mg OD till INR is between 2-3). Continue treatment for 6 weeks for post-surgical patients; lifelong if underlying predisposing factor (e.g. malignancy, etc.).
PE: low molecular weight heparin (Enoxaparin) 1.5 mg/kg (150 units/kg) OD + Warfarin 10 mg OD till INR is between 2-3. Stop Enoxaparin and continue Warfarin for 12 weeks for post-surgical patient; lifelong if underlying predisposing factor (e.g. malignancy).

Thrombo-embolic prophylaxis.
Low-risk patients: age <40, minor surgery (lasting <30 min) and no additional risk factors: no specific measures to prevent DVT are required other than early mobilization. Increasing age and duration of surgery increases risk of VTE.

High-risk patients: major surgery (lasting >30 min) who are aged >60. Prophylaxis measures: early mobilization. Above-knee thromboembolic stockings (AK-TEDs). Subcutaneous Heparin (low-dose non-fractioned Heparin LDUH or low molecular weight Heparin

LMWH). Enoxaparin 40 mg S/C OD. Intermittent pneumatic calf compression (IPC) boots, which are placed around the calves, are intermittently inflated and deflated, thereby increasing the flow of blood in calf veins (Fig. 6.7). At least a similar increase in calf veins blood flow can be achieved by popliteal nerve stimulation with the Geko® device (Fig. 6.8) which does not interfere with patient walking.

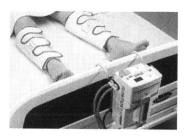

Fig. 6.7. Intermittent pneumatic compression calf pump.

Fig. 6.8. Illustration of the Geko® device for peroneal nerve stimulation.

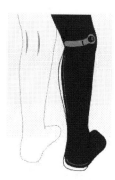

C. Balanced fluid replacement.
IV fluid prescription: daily fluid requirement can be calculated according to patient weight:
- For the first 10kg: 100ml/kg per 24h.
- For the next 10kg: 50ml/kg per 24h.
- For every kg above 20kg: 20ml/kg per 24h.
- 100 mmol of sodium and 70 mmol of potassium per 24h.

Thus a patient who is 70 kg will need 2500 ml of fluids. This includes 1L of normal saline and 1.5L of 5% dextrose, with 20mmol of potassium.

D. Positional and surgical access complications.
Unavoidable tissue damage to nerves or muscles may occur during many types of surgery (e.g., erectile dysfunction or incontinence following prostate surgery). There is also a risk of injury whilst under

general anaesthetic and being transported and handled in the theatre. These include injuries due to falls from the trolley, damage to diseased bones and joints during positioning, nerve palsies and diathermy burns.

Incisional hernia.
Occurs in 10-15% of abdominal wounds, usually appearing within the first year after surgery. Risk factors include obesity, poor muscle tone, wound infection and multiple uses of the same incision (re-operations).

Wound dehiscence.
About 2% of midline laparotomy wounds. Predisposing factors: poor blood supply, suture tension, long-term steroids, radiotherapy and malnutrition. It has a mortality rate of up to 30%. It is mainly due to failure of the wound closure technique. It usually occurs between 7 and 10 days postoperatively. It may be preceded by blood stained discharge from the wound. Initial management includes analgesia, sterile dressing, fluid resuscitation and early return to theatre for closure.

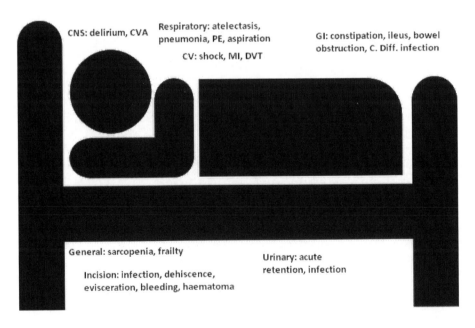

Fig. 6.9. Possible generic post-operative complications.

2. **Procedure specific post-operative complications.**

A. Cystoscopy.

Indications: haematuria, marked frequency and urgency, dysuria, recurrent or complicated UTIs, urethral or intravesical pathology suspected (e.g. carcinoma in situ, bladder stone), follow-up surveillance of patients with previously diagnosed bladder cancer. Fig. 6.10.

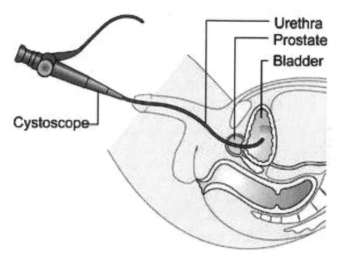

Fig. 6.10. Flexible cystoscopy diagram.

Complications:
a) Mild burning or bleeding on passing urine for a short period after procedure. No treatment needed, just reassure.
b) Infection, treat with antibiotics.
c) Urethral stricture: needs elective assessment.
d) Very rarely, perforation of the bladder, with or without peritonitis.

B. TURP.

Indications: LUTS, recurrent acute urinary retention, renal impairment due to bladder outlet obstruction, recurrent haematuria due to benign prostatic enlargement, bladder stones. Any complication of an enlarged prostate. Obstruction in prostate cancer. Fig. 6.11.

Fig. 6.11.
TURP
diagram.

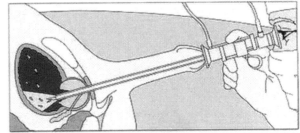

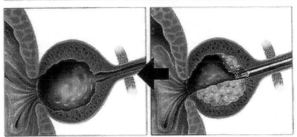

Complications:
a) Temporary mild burning on passing urine.
b) Urinary frequency.
c) Retrograde ejaculation in 75% of patients. This may produce infertility.
d) Failure of symptom resolution.
e) Sexual dysfunction.
f) UTI requiring antibiotic therapy.
g) Re-growth, 10% of patients require re-do surgery for recurrent prostatic obstruction (usually after years of the first TURP).
h) Failure to pass urine after the post-operative catheter has been removed, usually due to detrusor failure.
i) Urethral stricture formation.
j) Incontinence.
k) Absorption of irrigating fluid causing confusion and heart failure (TUR syndrome).
l) Very rarely, perforation of the bladder.
m) Catheter blockage: by a blood clot or by a chip of prostate left in the bladder during the operation. Symptoms: the bladder will be painfully distended. The irrigation flow will have stopped. Treatment: bladder washouts; if it fails attach a bladder syringe to the end of the catheter and pull back. Suck out the clot or chip of prostate and flow may restart. If it does not, change the catheter. If the bladder is full with clots, take the patient back to the theatre.

n) Haemorrhage: minor bleeding after TURP (rosé wine) is common and will stop spontaneously, requires no action. A dark red wine (moderate haematuria): increase the flow of irrigation and apply gentle traction to the catheter (with the balloon inflated), thereby pulling it onto the bladder neck or into the prostatic fossa to tamponade bleeding for 20 min or so. This will usually result in the urine clearing. Frank blood (bright red bleeding, suggesting serious haemorrhage): traction of the catheter can be tried, but at the same time you should make preparations to return the patient to theatre because it is unlikely that bleeding of this degree will stop. Post-operative bleeding requiring a return to theatre occurs in ~0.5% of cases.

C. TURBT.

Indications: tissue diagnosis of bladder tumours, local control of non-muscle-invasive bladder cancer (i.e. stops bleeding from tumours), staging of bladder cancer. Fig. 6.12.

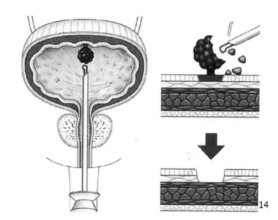

Fig. 6.12. TURBT diagram.

Complications:
a) Mild burning on passing urine.
b) Additional treatment (intravesical chemotherapy or immunotherapy) usually given to reduce the risk of future tumour recurrence.
c) UTI: treat with antibiotics.
d) Delayed bleeding: irrigate as per TURP or re-operate.
e) Development of a urethral stricture.
f) Bladder perforation.

D. Optical urethrotomy.

Indications: bulbar and penile urethral strictures. Fig. 6.13.

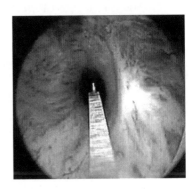

Fig. 6.13. Internal endoscopic urethrotomy. Sachse blade in urethral lumen.

Complications:
a) Mild burning on passing urine for short periods after the operation.
b) Optional self-catheterization to keep the stricture from closing down again.
c) UTI: treat with antibiotics.
d) Recurrence of stricture.
e) Sexual dysfunction.

E. Circumcision.

Indications (medical): phimosis, paraphimosis, penile cancer biopsy or treatment, any foreskin lesion requiring histology, recurrent balanitis, functional (coital) phimosis or paraphimosis, failure of other treatments (creams, dilatations, preputioplasty). Fig. 6.14.

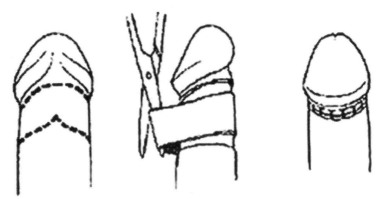

Fig. 6.14. Circumcision diagram.

Complications:

a) Haemorrhage: apply pressure dressing; if it doesn't stop suture the bleeding vessel under local anaesthesia.
b) Necrosis of the skin of the shaft of the penis: wait for the necrotic tissue to demarcate before assessing the extent of the problem. The penis has a superb blood supply and has remarkable healing characteristics.
c) Separation of the skin of the coronal sulcus from the shaft skin: if limited to a small area this will heal spontaneously. If a larger circumference of the wound has dehisced, re-suture in theatre.
d) Wound infection: local antisepsis and dressings. Antibiotics if temperature or immune compromise.
e) Urethro-cutaneous fistula or urethral damage (i.e. due to a stitch placed through the urethra): it will need delayed correction.
f) Excessive removal of skin: re-epithelialization can occur if the defect between the glans and the shaft skin is not large. If the defect is large, the end result will be a buried penis (the glans retracts towards the skin at the base of the penis). Will need reconstructive re-operation.
g) Permanent altered sensation of the penis.
h) Persistence of absorbable stitches: just wait.
i) Scar tenderness, rarely long-term.
j) Poor cosmetics: it may rarely need revision (cosmetic). Occasional need for removal of excessive skin at a later date.

F. Hydrocoele and epididymal cyst removal.
Indications: large or symptomatic hydrocele. Large or painful epididymal cyst. Fig. 6.15.

Hydrocoele aspiration: strict attention to antisepsis is vital, since introduction of infection into a closed space leads to abscess formation. Avoid superficial blood vessels (if you hit them, a large haematoma can result). Recurrence is the rule, so try to stay clear of problems and try not to aspirate, it creates a thicker tunica and makes the likely unavoidable operation more difficult.

Hydrocoele resection and Epididymal cyst removal: avoid in young men who wish to maintain fertility, since epididymal obstruction can occur.

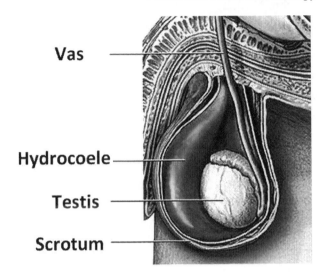

Vas

Hydrocoele

Testis

Scrotum

Fig. 6.15.
Hydrocele
diagram.

Complications:
a) Scrotal swelling: resolves spontaneously but it may take several weeks.
b) Haematoma formation: RICE (rest, ice, compression -mild-, elevation).
c) Hydrocoele recurrence: only happens if tunica is preserved, so use a technique with tunica resection or eversion.
d) Infection: liberal use of antibiotics. If abscess, drain it first.

G. Nesbitt's procedure.
Indications: Peyronie's disease, congenital curvature. Fig. 6.16.

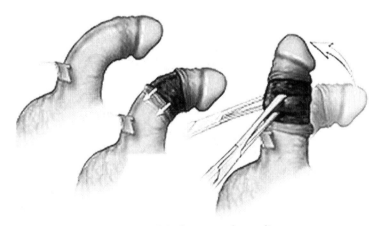

Fig. 6.16. Nesbitt's procedure diagram.

Complications:
a) Penile shortening.
b) Poor cosmetics.
c) Temporary swelling and bruising of the penis and scrotum.
d) Partial correction of the bend.
e) Bleeding (manage as circumcision) or infection (treat).
f) Sexual dysfunction.
g) Penile dysesthesia.

H. Vasectomy.
Indications: permanent birth control, usually irreversible. Fig. 6.17.

Complications:
a) Haematoma can occur: RICE.
b) Failure to identify vas at the time of surgery and not ligated (or, very rarely, that there were 2 vas deferens on one side). The control sperm count will show failure.
c) The vas deferens can re-canalize, thereby restoring fertility and pregnancy (1 in 2000).
d) Sperm granuloma, a hard, pea-sized sometimes painful lump in the region of the cut ends of the vas. It can be a cause of chronic pain, in which case it may have to be excised.
e) Inflammation or infection of testes or epididymis, requiring antibiotics.

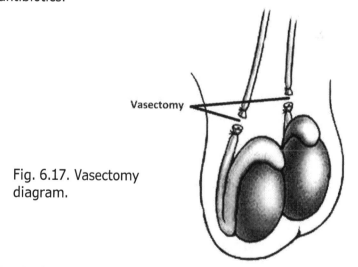

Fig. 6.17. Vasectomy
diagram.

I. Orchiectomy.
Indications: radical (inguinal) orchiectomy for excision of testis with a

suspected tumour. Simple orchiectomy (bilateral): for testosterone suppression to control advanced prostate cancer. Done via a scrotal approach.

Complications:
a) Scrotal haematoma: drain it if large or enlarging or if there are signs of infection (fever, discharge of pus from the wound). RICE.
b) Infection: fever, discharge of pus from the wound, abscess. Antibiotics for 3 to 4 weeks. Drain if an abscess is present.
c) For radical orchiectomy: damage to the ilio-inguinal nerve leading to an area of loss of sensation overlying the scrotum.
d) Infertility.
e) Infection of the incision may occur, requiring further treatment and possibly removal of implant if one has been inserted.
f) Pain requiring removal of implant if this has been inserted.
g) Cosmetic expectation not always met.

J. JJ Stent.

Indications (see also renal colic chapter 2.4): relief of obstruction from ureteric stones, clots or ureteric strictures. Prevention of obstruction: post ureteroscopy. Passive dilatation of ureter prior to ureteroscopy. To ensure antegrade flow of urine following surgery (e.g. pyeloplasty) or injury to ureter. Following endopyelotomy.

Complications:
a) Suprapubic pain.
b) LUTS (frequency, urgency, as the stent irritates trigone). consider using anticholinergics.
c) Haematuria: increase diuresis.
d) Urinary tract infection: in case of sepsis place a urethral catheter to lower the pressure in the collecting system and prevent reflux of infected urine. Treat with IV antibiotics.
e) Incorrect placement (buckled or distal end into the ureter): endoscopic re-positioning under X rays.
f) Stent migration (up the ureter is rare, or down the ureter and into bladder): replace.
g) Stent blockage: re-operate.
h) If not removed or changed when due, it becomes encrusted with stones, and removal may be very difficult.

K. Nephrectomy and Nephro-ureterectomy.

Nephrectomy.
Indications: renal cell cancer, non-functioning kidney with or without a calculus, persistent haemorrhage following renal trauma. Persistent or progressive sepsis in spite of drainage and antibiotics.

Nephro-ureterectomy.
Indications: upper urinary tract urothelial cancer. Refluxing atrophic kidney.

Complications (both):
a) Haemorrhage: from the renal pedicle or the spleen. Symptoms: tachycardia, cold periphery, falling urine output, and eventually a drop in blood pressure (hypovolemic shock). Check the drain but it may still be negative. May need further surgery and/or transfusion. Escalate care and contact the performing surgical team.
b) Wound infection: if superficial, treat with antibiotics. If an underlying collection of pus is suspected, open the wound to allow free drainage, and pack daily.
c) Pancreatic injury. Signs: excessive drainage of fluid from the drain, with a high amylase level. If no drain is present, an abdominal collection will develop, which may be manifested by a prolonged ileus. May need re-operation. Contact surgical team. CT is usually diagnostic.
d) Pneumothorax (diaphragm lesion) is rare. It may need drainage.
e) Renal failure: if suspected, contact renal support team. The patient may need hemofiltration for a period. Eventually the nephrologist may need to be involved.
f) Involvement or injury to nearby structures or blood vessels, spleen, lung, liver, pancreas, bowel (look for peritonitis): it will probably need a CT for diagnosis, and a General Surgery input.
g) Infection, pain, or hernia of incision.
h) Anaesthetic or cardiovascular problems, (including chest infection, pulmonary embolus, CVA, deep vein thrombosis, heart attack). As any general anaesthetic.

L. Radical prostatectomy.
Indications: localized prostate cancer. Fig. 6.18.

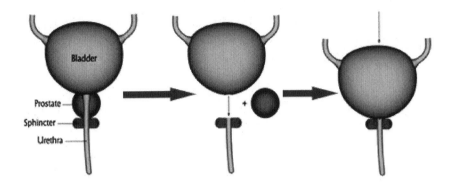

Fig. 6.18. Radical prostatectomy diagram.

Complications:
a) Persistent leak of fluid from the drains: send a sample for urea and creatinine, and if it is urine (not lymph), get a cystogram to determine the size of the leak at the vesico-urethral junction.
b) Haemorrhage: managed in the usual way (transfusion; return to theatre where bleeding persists or where there is cardiovascular compromise).
c) Ureteric obstruction: usually results from oedema of the bladder, arrange placement of percutaneous nephrostomy.
d) Lymphocele: drain; or open to the peritoneum from which it is absorbed.
e) Urethral catheter malfunction and loss: if out a week after surgery, the patient may void successfully. If it falls out early after surgery, the surgical team may gently attempt to replace it with a 12Fr catheter which has been well lubricated. If this fails, an endoscopic assessment is needed. If the patient is unable to void, after catheter removal, a suprapubic catheter can be placed (percutaneous, or under general anaesthetic via an open cystostomy).
f) Faecal fistula: due to rectal injury. Formal closure is required by the colorectal team.
g) Vesico-urethral anastomosis stricture: gentle dilatation may be tried. If the stricture recurs, instruct the patient in ISD, in an attempt to keep the stricture open. If this fails, bladder neck incision may be tried.
h) High chance of erectile dysfunction due to unavoidable nerve damage. Early penile rehabilitation should be offered. Can

improve during the 1st postoperative year.

i) No semen is produced, causing infertility.

j) Urinary incontinence: temporary or permanent, requiring pads or further surgery. Can also improve during the 1st postoperative year.

k) Cancer treatment at a later date may be required, particularly if follow up PSAs start rising.

l) Anaesthetic or cardiovascular problems (including chest infection, pulmonary embolus, CVA, deep vein thrombosis, heart attack).

m) Pain, infection, or hernia in area of incision.

M. Radical cystectomy.

Indications: muscle-invasive bladder cancer, non-muscle-invasive bladder cancer which has failed to respond to intravesical chemotherapy or immunotherapy, recurrent bladder cancer post radiotherapy (Fig. 6.19). Interstitial cystitis and refractory incontinence or fistula may rarely need cystectomy.

Fig. 6.19. Cystectomy diagram. Bladder (B), ureters (U) and colon (C).

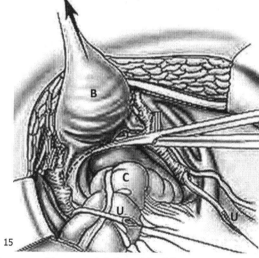

Combined with urethrectomy if: multiple bladder tumours, involvement of bladder neck or urethra.

Complications:

a) Haemorrhage: persistent bleeding which fails to respond to transfusion should be managed by re-exploration.

b) Wound dehiscence: requires re-suturing under general anaesthetic.

c) Ileus: common. Usually resolves spontaneously within a few days.

May need NGT.

d) Small bowel obstruction: continue nasogastric aspiration. The obstruction will usually resolve spontaneously. Re-operation is occasionally required where the obstruction persists or where there are signs of bowel ischaemia.

e) Leakage from the intestinal anastomosis: peritonitis requires re-operation and repair, or refashioning of the anastomosis. Entero-cutaneous fistula: bowel contents leak from the intestine and through a fistulous track onto the skin. If low-volume leak (<500ml/24h), will usually heal spontaneously. Normal (enteral) nutrition may be maintained until the fistula closes (which usually occurs within a matter of days or a few weeks). If high-volume, spontaneous closure is less likely and re-operation to close the fistula may be required. Always involve the surgical team **early**.

f) Pelvic abscess: formal surgical (open) exploration of the pelvis is indicated with drainage of the abscess and careful inspection to see if the underlying cause is a rectal injury, in which case a colostomy should be performed.

g) Sexual dysfunction. Early penile rehabilitation should be offered. Can improve during the 1st postoperative year.

h) No semen is produced, causing infertility.

i) Pain or difficulty with sexual intercourse in females, due to narrowing or shortening of vagina (if preserved) and need for removal of uterus and ovaries.

j) Infection or hernia of incision.

k) Anaesthetic or cardiovascular problems (including chest infection, pulmonary embolus, CVA, deep vein thrombosis, heart attack).

l) Decreased renal function with time.

m) Rectal injury.

n) Shortened bowel, producing diarrhoea and vitamin absorption deficiency requiring treatment.

o) Urine fistula: it must be thoroughly evaluated and may require elective re-operation.

p) Stricture of bowel or ureters.

q) Scarring, narrowing, or hernia formation around stoma opening, requiring revision.

N. Ileal conduit.

Indications: urinary diversion following radical cystectomy, intractable incontinence for which anti-incontinence surgery has failed or is not appropriate. Fig. 6.20.

Fig. 6.20. Ileal
conduit diagram.
Kidneys (K),
ureters (U), ileal
conduit (I).

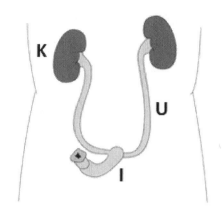

Complications:
a) Ileus, small bowel obstruction and leakage from the intestinal anastomosis (as in cystectomy above).
b) Leakage from the uretero-ileal anastomosis: suspected with a persistently high output of fluid from the drain. Test fluid for urea. Urine will have a higher urea and creatinine concentration than serum. If the fluid is lymph or peritoneal fluid, the urea and creatinine concentration will be the same as that of serum. Arrange a loop-gram (conduit-gram). This will confirm the leak. Place a soft, small catheter (12Ch) into the conduit to encourage antegrade flow of urine and assist healing of the uretero-ileal anastomosis. If the leakage continues, nephrostomies for diversion may be needed, or antegrade JJ re-stenting. Occasionally, an uretero-ileal leak will present as an urinoma (this causes a persistent ileus). Radiological drain insertion can resolve it.
c) Hyper-chloraemic acidosis: due to urine absorption in the conduit. May be associated with obstruction of the stoma at its distal end or from infrequent emptying of the bag. Catheterize the stoma. In the long term, the conduit may have to be surgically shortened.
d) Acute pyelonephritis: due to the presence of reflux combined with bacteriuria.
e) Stoma stenosis: the distal (cutaneous) end of the stoma may become narrowed, usually as a result of ischaemia to the distal part of the conduit. Revision surgery is required if this stenosis causes obstruction leading to recurrent UTIs or upper tract dilatation.
f) Para-stoma hernia formation: around the site through which the

conduit passes, through the fascia of the anterior abdominal wall. ~30% incidence. Some hernias can be left alone. The indications for repairing a hernia are: bowel obstruction, pain, difficulty with applying the stoma bag (distortion of the skin around the stoma by the hernia can lead to frequent bag detachment).

g) Urinary infections.
h) Diarrhoea due to shortened bowel.
i) Bleeding.
j) Infection or hernia of incision.
k) Stricture to bowel or ureters.
l) Decreased renal function with time.

O. Percutaneous nephrolithotomy (PCNL).

Indications: renal or upper ureter stones >1.5 cm in diameter, stones that have failed ESWL and/or an attempt at flexible ureteroscopy and laser treatment, staghorn calculi. Fig. 6.21.

Fig. 6.21. PCNL diagram.

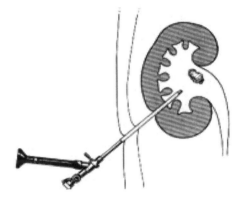

Complications:
a) Bleeding: if persistent and severe, transfusion, embolization, or, at last resort, surgical removal of kidney is needed.
b) Septicaemia.
c) Colonic perforation: look for peritonitis or faecal content around the nephrostomy.
d) Damage to the liver or spleen: look for peritonitis or shock.
e) Damage to the lung and pleura leading to pneumothorax or pleural effusion.
f) Nephro-cutaneous fistula: particularly if ureter is obstructed.
g) Failure to remove all stones.
h) Over absorption of irrigating fluids into the blood: mainly intra-

operative, and it creates hypervolemia with all its consequences.

P. Ureteroscopy.

Indications: stones, typically in the distal or middle ureter that are unlikely to pass spontaneously or are causing significant discomfort, stones in the kidney that are not treatable by SWL. As an investigation to determine the reason for blood in the urine or positive cytology. Endoscopic management of upper tract urothelial carcinoma. Fig. 6.22.

Complications:
a) Ureteric perforation or avulsion.
b) Mild burning or bleeding on passing urine for a short period after the operation.

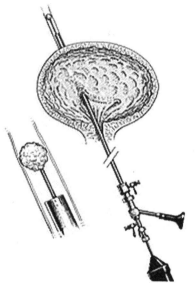

Fig. 6.22. Ureteroscopy diagram and close up.

c) Urinary infections.
d) Inability to get to the stone or movement of stone back into kidney where it is not retrievable.
e) Kidney damage or infection.
f) Failure to pass scope if ureter is narrow.
g) Recurrence of stones.
h) Ureteric stricture (<3%).

Q. Pyeloplasty.

Indications: PUJ (pelvic-ureteric-junction) obstruction. Fig. 6.23.

Complications:
a) Haemorrhage.
b) Urinary leak: if a urethral catheter has not been left in place, catheterize the patient to minimize bladder pressure and therefore the chance of reflux, which might be responsible for the leak.

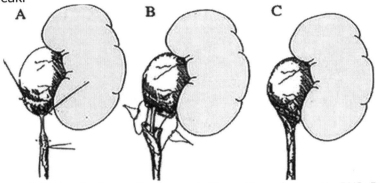

Fig. 6.23. Pyeloplasty diagram. A. Resection of stenotic PUJ. B. Spatulation of ureter over a stent. C. Pyelo-ureteral anastomosis.

c) Recurrence.
d) Acute pyelonephritis.
e) Entry into lung cavity.
f) Anaesthetic or cardiovascular problems (including chest infection, pulmonary embolus, CVA, deep vein thrombosis, heart attack).
g) Need to remove kidney at a later time.
h) Infection, pain, or hernia of incision.

R. Scrotal exploration for torsion and orchidopexy.

Indications: suspected testicular torsion. Fig. 6.24.

Fig. 6.24. Diagram of testicular torsion (torsion of the spermatic cord).

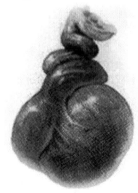

Complications:
a) Scrotal hematoma.
b) Possible infection of incision, or of the testis.
c) Testicular atrophy.
d) Infertility.

S. Endoscopic cysto-lithotomy (lithotripsy) and (open) cysto-litholapaxy.

To clarify terms: lithos = stone, tripsis = to rub or pound, lapaxis = emptying out, tome from temnein = to cut (all from Greek). Lithotomy and lithotripsy imply fragmenting the stone. Litholapaxy implies removing it without fragmentation. These terms are frequently used interchangeably.

Indications: endoscopic cystolithotomy generally indicated for bladder stones <6cm in diameter. Open cystolitholapaxy (Fig. 6.25) for stones >6cm in diameter or patients with urethral obstruction which precludes adequate endoscopic access to the bladder.

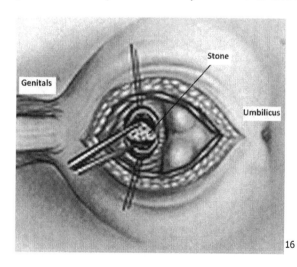

Fig. 6.25. Diagram of open cystolitholapaxy.

Complications:
a) Haematuria.
b) Septicaemia.
c) Bladder perforation (with endoscopic approach).
d) Mild burning or bleeding on passing urine after the operation.
e) Recurrence of stones or residual stone fragments.
f) Injury to urethra causing stricture.

T. Laparoscopic surgery.

General advantages over open surgery: reduced post-operative pain, smaller scars (better cosmetics, less incisional hernias), less disturbance of bowel function (less post-operative ileus), reduced recovery time, earlier return to normal daily life activities, reduced hospital stay, generally reduced costs (when all aspects considered).

General contraindications to laparoscopic surgery:
1. Severe COPD (use of pressured CO_2 for insufflation).
2. Non correctable coagulopathy, as manoeuvres to secure haemostasis may be slower or more difficult to implement.
3. Abdominal wall infection.
4. Massive haemo-peritoneum.
5. Generalized peritonitis.
6. Suspected malignant ascites.
7. Infected organs, as additional pressure increases bacteraemia.

Complications:
a) Gas embolism (potentially fatal).
b) Hypercarbia.
c) Subcutaneous emphysema.
d) Pneumothorax, pneumo-mediastinum and pneumo-pericardium.
e) During port access, there might be bowel, vessels, anterior abdominal wall and viscus injury.
f) Post-operatively, bowel may become entrapped in the trocar sites (incisional hernia), or there may be bleeding from that point.
g) Temporary shoulder tip pain.
h) Temporary abdominal bloating.
i) Infection or pain of incision.
j) Haemorrhage.
k) Conversion to open surgery.
l) Recognized (and unrecognized) injury to organs or blood vessels requiring correction.
m) Anaesthetic or cardiovascular problems (including chest infection, pulmonary embolus, CVA, deep vein thrombosis, MI).

Many complications of laparoscopy are avoided or reduced by a retro or sub-peritoneal approach.

U. Prostate Biopsy.

Indications: confirmed high PSA level for age or a suspicious DRE.

Previous biopsies showing PIN or ASAP. Previous biopsies normal, but PSA rising or DRE becoming suspicious. Fig. 6.26.

Complications:
If a systemic infection is found, resuscitate the patient, escalate to ITU if necessary, and give I/V antibiotics including: Gentamycin, Metronidazole and Penicillin. Don't waste time, and have the courtesy of informing the performing team.

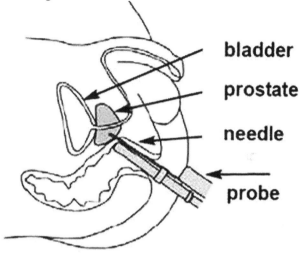

Fig. 6.26. Trans-rectal prostate biopsy diagram.

Complication type	%
Haematospermia	37.4
Haematuria > 1 day	14.5
Rectal bleeding < 2 days	2.2
Prostatitis	1.0
Septicaemia	0.8
Epididymitis	0.7
Rectal bleeding > 2 days ± requiring surgical intervention	0.7
Urinary retention	0.2
Other complications requiring hospitalization	0.3

V. Acute renal transplant rejection.

Renal transplantation is the best treatment for patients with end stage renal failure. It improves the quality of life and prognosis of these patients. Acute rejection is one of the possible complications and it happens due to the genetic differences between donor and receptor and other factors like ischaemia time. New immunosuppressant are effective, so this complication is present in 10-20% of recipients. An early diagnosis of rejection can improve management outcomes.

Aetiology:
- T cell mediated rejection.
- Acute rejection mediated by antibodies.
- Subclinical rejection seen in biopsies.

Classification:
- Hyperacute rejection: happens almost immediately after the vascular anastomosis. Due to anti-HLA or anti-AB antibodies. Infrequent. The transplanted organ is lost. It is an intra-operative complication most of the times.
- Transplant rupture: pain at implant site, palpable enlarged implant, hypotension or shock.
- Acute rejection: frequent. After postoperative day 5 and before 3-6 months. Reduced urine output, haematuria, general malaise, temperature, pain at implant site.

Treatment.
Medical. Maximal immunosuppressant management by the nephrology team. Usually a biopsy is done before treatment. Most protocols use calcineurin inhibitors (Cyclosporine A or Tacrolimus), steroids and nucleotides synthesis inhibitors (Azathioprine, Mofetil Mycophenolate).

Surgical. Transplantectomy for non-functional implants with symptoms. Elective if possible.

Additional reading:
1. Anticoagulation and Antiplatelet Therapy in Urologic Practice: ICUD and AUA Review Paper. American Urological Association. https://www.auanet.org/common/pdf/education/clinical-guidance/Anticoagulation-Antiplatelet-Therapy.pdf. On 02/04/2016.
2. The geko™ electro-stimulation device for venous thromboembolism prophylaxis: a

NICE medical technology guidance. Summers JA, Clinch J, Radhakrishnan M, Healy A, McMillan V, Morris E, Rua T, Ofuya M, Wang Y, Dimmock PW, Lewis C, Peacock JL, Keevil SF. Appl Health Econ Health Policy. 2015 Apr; 13(2): 135-47.

3. The effectiveness of a novel neuromuscular electrostimulation method versus intermittent pneumatic compression in enhancing lower limb blood flow. Jawad H, Bain DS, Dawson H, Crawford K, Johnston A, Tucker A. J Vasc Surg Venous Lymphat Disord. 2014 Apr; 2(2): 160-5.

4. Reporting and grading of complications after urologic surgical procedures: an ad hoc EAU guidelines panel assessment and recommendations. Mitropoulos D, Artibani W, Graefen M, Remzi M, Rouprêt M, Truss M; Asociación Europea de Urología. Actas Urol Esp. 2013 Jan; 37(1):1-11.

5. Patient Information Leaflets. The British Association of Urological Surgeons. http://www.baus.org.uk/patients/information_leaflets/. On 02/04/2016.

6. Classification of surgical complications: a new proposal with evaluation in a cohort of 6336 patients and results of a survey. Dindo D, Demartines N, Clavien PA. Ann Surg. 2004 Aug; 240(2): 205-13.

7. Best practice policy statement on urologic surgery antimicrobial prophylaxis. American Urological Association. https://www.auanet.org/common/pdf/education/clinical-guidance/Antimicrobial-Prophylaxis.pdf. On 02/04/2016.

8. Rejection of the kidney allograft. Nankivell BJ, Alexander SI. N Engl J Med. 2010 Oct 7; 363(15): 1451-62.

9. Endorsement of the Kidney Disease Improving Global Outcomes (KDIGO) guidelines on kidney transplantation: a European Renal Best Practice (ERBP) position statement. Heemann U, Abramowicz D, Spasovski G, Vanholder R. Nephrol Dial Transplant. 2011 Jul; 26(7): 2099-106.

10. EAU guidelines on renal transplantation. Kälble T, Lucan M, Nicita G, Sells R, Burgos Revilla FJ, Wiesel M. Eur Urol. 2005 Feb; 47(2): 156-66.

11. Transplantectomy following renal graft failure. Antón-Pérez G, Gallego-Samper R, Marrero-Robayna S, Henríquez-Palop F, Rodríguez-Pérez JC. Nefrologia. 2012; 32(5): 573-8.

12. Peritoneal approach to prosthetic mesh repair of paraostomy hernias. Sugarbaker PH. Ann Surg. 1985 Mar; 201(3): 344-6.

CHAPTER 7. Reno-vascular Emergencies.

7.1. Renal artery embolism.

Mr J Clavijo.

Definition.
It is the occlusion of the renal artery or of its branches by emboli. With stenosis and local thrombosis they make up the more frequent causes of renal artery obstruction and renal ischaemia. Segmental ischaemia leads to ischaemic necrosis of the affected area with consequent loss of function.

Aetiology.
The most frequent sources of emboli are atrial fibrillation, bacterial endocarditis, other valvular diseases, ischaemic cardiopathy and dilated cardio-myopathy.

Aortic and renal artery diseases can be sources of emboli on areas of abnormal endothelium (atherosclerosis, arterial by-pass thrombosis, arterial dissection, aneurism, arteritis, thrombosis associated with clotting disorders, arterial trauma, arterial compression). Endovascular studies or procedures.

Diagnosis.
1. History: variable and non-specific presentation. Loin or abdominal pain, acute and intense or colic, unilateral and persistent. Nausea, vomits, temperature, hypertension. Dyspepsia. Haematuria.

Past history: cardiovascular. Embolic episodes in other organs. Coagulopathy and/or cancer (prostate, pancreas, lung, renal). Medications.

2. Physical examination: rule out emboli in limbs and other organs. Temperature. Complete cardiovascular for AF and murmurs (endocarditis).

3. Investigations:
Blood: full coagulation screen. Blood culture if pyrexial. FBC. LFT. U&E. LDH will be high.

Image: angio-renal CT (Fig. 7.1) where the ischaemic area can be seen with a typical triangular distribution corresponding to the occluded branch (cone if 3D). Alternatively MRI.

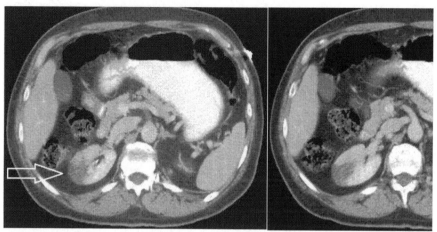

Fig. 7.1. CT shows right renal embolus and infarction (arrow).[17]

Arteriography (Fig. 7.2) is also diagnostic and allows for access to direct (in situ) thrombolysis.

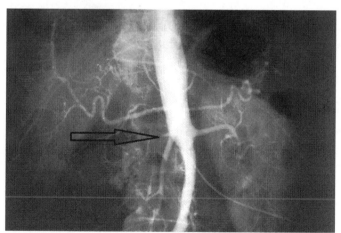

Fig. 7.2. Arteriogram with exclusion of right renal artery (arrow).

Echocardiogram for sources on emboli. Fig. 7.3.

Others: urine, MSU. ECG.

Treatment.

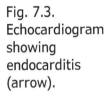

Fig. 7.3.
Echocardiogram
showing
endocarditis
(arrow).

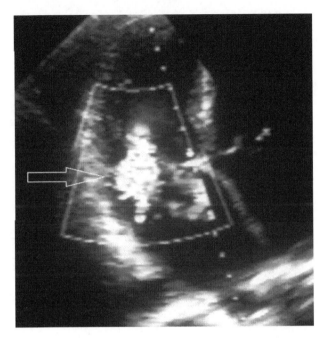

Medical: contact a cardiology and invasive radiology teams immediately. They will complete the diagnosis and treat the source of emboli and can organise in situ thrombolysis. Patent will need anticoagulation with heparin to prevent further emboli. In situ thrombolysis has better outcomes if done in the first 3 hours after pain started (infarction time). Just like testicular torsion, this is a time sensitive ischaemic emergency.

A nephrology consultation is prudent, and necessary if there is renal function compromise.

Surgical: a nephrectomy is rarely needed, particularly in the acute setting. Surgical reno-vascular removal of the embolus has comparable results to thrombolysis but higher morbidity and mortality.

Complications.
If the patient's renal function is compromised, the loss of renal mass can lead to different grades of renal failure. 30 day mortality is 11.4%.

Outcomes.

Will depend on residual renal function and the extension of the infarction area. Will be proportional to the response to treatment and how early and effectively it can be implemented.

Additional reading:

1. The clinical spectrum of acute renal infarction. Korzets Z, Plotkin E, Bernheim J, Zissin R. Isr Med Assoc J. 2002 Oct; 4(10): 781-4.
2. Acute renal artery embolism: a case report and brief literature review. Robinson S, Nichols D, Macleod A, Duncan J. Ann Vasc Surg. 2008 Jan; 22(1): 145-7.
3. Acute renal failure caused by renal artery embolism. Blasco Patiño F, Gómez Moreno J, Román García F, Martínez López de Letona J, Moar Martínez C. An Med Interna. 2002 Apr; 19(4): 210-2.
4. The significance of clinical features in the prognosis of acute renal infarction: single center experience. Rhee H, Song SH, Won Lee D, Lee SB, Kwak IS, Seong EY. Clin Exp Nephrol. 2012 Aug; 16(4): 611-6.
5. Renal artery embolism: a case report and review. Kansal S, Feldman M, Cooksey S, Patel S. J Gen Intern Med. 2008 May; 23(5): 644-7.
6. Renal artery occlusion. Wright MP, Persad RA, Cranston DW. BJU Int. 2001 Jan; 87(1): 9-12.
7. Local thrombolytic treatment for renal arterial embolism. Glück G, Croitoru M, Deleanu D, Platon P. Eur Urol. 2000 Sep; 38(3): 339-43.
8. Renal infarction in bacterial endocarditis diagnosed by computed tomography. Berliner L, Redmond P, DeBlasi J. Urol Radiol. 1982; 4(4): 231-3.

7.2. Renal vein thrombosis.

Mr J Clavijo.

Definition.
It is the occlusion of the renal vein or of its branches by thrombi. With stenosis (retro-aortic vein, aorta-mesenteric compression) is the most frequent cause of obstruction and raised renal vein pressure. This produces renal oedema, possibly nephrotic syndrome and collateral circulation amongst other problems.

Aetiology.
It's seen associated with IVC thrombosis, nephrotic syndrome, hypovolaemia, coagulopathies, kidney tumours and trauma.
Causes (Virchow's triad):
1. Endothelial damage: direct trauma, trauma during venography, renal transplant, tumour infiltration, acute rejection, vasculitis, homocystinuria.
2. Stasis: severe volume loss, significant bleeding, dehydration, post-transplant, retroperitoneal tumours compressing the renal vein, vascular crossings.
3. Hypercoagulability: nephrotic syndrome, membranous glomerulonephritis, membranous proliferative glomerulonephritis, glomerulosclerosis, sepsis, puerperal, disseminated cancers, oral contraceptives, factor V Leiden (activated protein C resistance), prothrombin gene mutation, protein S deficiency, protein C deficiency, anti-thrombin deficiency, anti-phospholipid syndrome, lupus, Behcet disease, AIDS nephropathy.

Classification.
- Acute, that may present with symptoms.
- Gradual. Generally asymptomatic due to compensatory collateral circulation.

Diagnosis.
1. History: haematuria, loin pain, palpable mass (in neonates and small children), reduced split function of the compromised kidney. This is the acute presentation, which is the least frequent. More often it is completely asymptomatic.
Past history: anything predisposing to thrombosis. Endovascular

procedures. Medications: anticoagulants and why they're used.

2. Physical examination: look for predisposing factors. Subcutaneous collateral circulation. Enlarged kidney.

3. Investigations:
Blood: FBC. Coagulation screen. LFT. U&Es.

Image: USS is the preferred initial investigation. It will show an increase in renal size, reduced echogenicity due to oedema, absence of venous flow.

CT is diagnostic and can localize the extension of the thrombus and show collateral veins (Fig. 7.4). MRI has more sensitivity and specificity (Fig. 7.5).

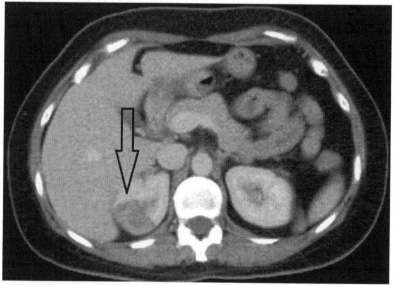

Fig. 7.4. CT shows segmental right renal vein thrombosis (arrow).[18]

Other: urine dip.

Treatment.
Medical: regardless of aetiology anticoagulation is the basis of treatment, particularly in the acute setting. In situ, trans catheter thrombolysis is an alternative for selected patients with acute renal vein thrombosis. This can be considered in patients with acute onset

of symptoms and renal dysfunction with no contraindication to systemic thrombolytic agents.

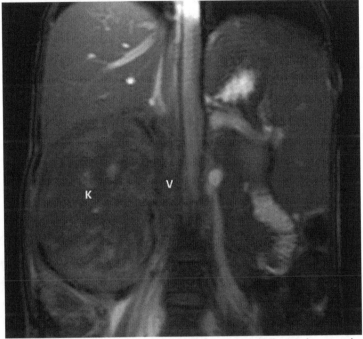

Fig. 7.5. MRI shows right renal enlargement (K). Right renal vein thrombosis advancing into IVC (V).[19]

Indications of thrombectomy/thrombolysis: failure of adequate anticoagulation, complications (PE), bilateral thrombosis, acute renal failure, thrombosis n single kidney, extension into IVC, contraindication for systemic anticoagulation, renal transplant, severe persistent pain.

Surgical: thrombectomy does not produce dramatic results. It should be considered in the unusual case of bilateral thrombosis and renal failure unresponsive to anticoagulation. Surgery does not prevent recurrence.

Any predisposing factors should be rapidly and effectively addressed.

Complications.
The thrombotic process can advance into the IVC and produce PE and death. Bilateral compromise can produce renal failure and

hypertension.

Outcomes.

They are proportional to the response to anticoagulation.

Prognostic factors: baseline renal function, contralateral kidney function, slow progression, adequate collateral veins drainage, adequate treatment, severity and progression of predisposing conditions.

Additional reading:

1. Successful treatment of acute inferior vena cava and unilateral renal vein thrombosis by local infusion of recombinant tissue plasminogen activator. Lam KK, Lui CC. Am J Kidney Dis. 1998 Dec; 32(6): 1075-9.
2. Renal vein occlusion: diagnosis and treatment. Witz M, Korzets Z. Isr Med Assoc J. 2007 May; 9(5): 402-5.
3. Renal vein thrombosis. Asghar M, Ahmed K, Shah SS, Siddique MK, Dasgupta P, Khan MS. Eur J Vasc Endovasc Surg. 2007 Aug; 34(2): 217-23.

7.3. Non traumatic retroperitoneal haematoma.

Mr J Clavijo.

Definition.
It is the spontaneous collection of blood or clots in the retroperitoneal space in the absence of significant trauma.

Aetiology.
This is a rare condition. The usual causes are a ruptured abdominal aortic aneurism, and spontaneous bleeding from renal tumours (Wunderlich syndrome), mainly renal cell carcinomas and angiomyolipomata. More rarely rupture of: adrenal tumours, renal artery aneurysms, arteritis, congenital arterio-venous malformations and cysts. Other infrequent causes are uretero-arterial fistulas and coagulation disorders.

Classification.
According to the organ of origin (renal, vascular, and adrenal).

Diagnosis.
1. History: presentation can be insidious and challenging. It may present with haemodynamic compromise, loin pain or palpable mass or a combination of them. Can also be found on radiological assessment for non-specific symptoms (CT, USS).

Past medical history: AAA, urological conditions, haematuria. Tuberous sclerosis, where AMLs tend to be larger and rupture more. Von Recklinghausen, for phaeochromocytomas. Bleeding disorders. Pregnancy. Radiotherapy. AMLs or RCCs on active surveillance. Drug history: anticoagulation, anti-platelets.

2. Physical examination: palpable flank mass. Haematuria. Loin pain. Adrenal failure (Addisonian crisis).

3. Investigations:
Blood: FBC, coagulation screen, renal function. Group/cross match blood. ESR/CRP, glucose, amylase, calcium.

Imaging:
CT scan of abdomen with contrast. Fig. 7.6 and 7.7.

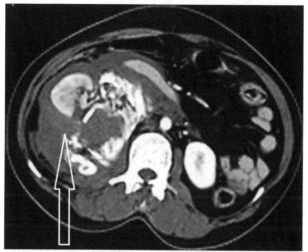

Fig. 7.6. Right retro-peritoneal haematoma (arrow).

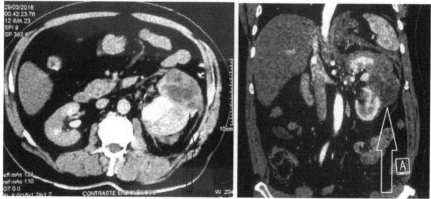

Fig. 7.7. Left retro-peritoneal haematoma. Ruptured renal tumour (arrows).

In selected cases angiography, particularly if arterial origin is suspected and embolization is considered (significant co-morbidities). It can be both diagnostic and therapeutic. Fig. 7.8.

Others: urine pregnancy test.

Treatment.
Medical.

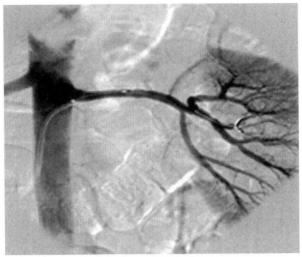
Fig. 7.8. Renal arteriogram.

Diagnosed and managed in a similar way to a renal blunt trauma. Standard resuscitation and trauma protocol applies.

Surgical.
Once the patient is stable and the haematoma is re-absorbed, the underlying condition (cause) can be electively managed in the usual way, consider surgery if appropriate.

Only explore in an acute situation if patient rapidly deteriorating in spite of adequate resuscitation. In aortic or iliac artery bleedings, early involvement of a vascular surgeon is vital.

Complications.
Acute hypovolemia and shock. Delayed ones: retroperitoneal fibrosis, Page's kidney (peri-renal fibrosis producing hypertension).

Outcomes.
These will depend on the response to resuscitation and to definitive treatment of each causative pathology.

Additional reading:
1. Urological Trauma. European Association of Urology Guidelines. http://uroweb.org/wp-content/uploads/EAU-Guidelines-Urological-Trauma-2015-v2.pdf. On 04/04/2016.
2. Imaging of renal trauma: a comprehensive review. Kawashima A, Sandler CM, Corl FM, West OC, Tamm EP, Fishman EK, Goldman SM. Radiographics. 2001. May-Jun;

21(3): 557-74.

3.   Retroperitoneal and upper tract haemorrhage. Rajpurkar AD, Santucci RA. In: Urological Emergencies. A practical Guide. Wessells H, McAninch JW. New Jersey: Humana Press; 2005. p 181.

4.   Spontaneous retroperitoneal haemorrhage of renal origin (Wunderlich syndrome): analysis of 8 cases. Molina Escudero R, Castillo OA. Arch Esp Urol. 2013 Dec; 66(10): 925-9.

CHAPTER 8. Urology Related Hypertensive Crisis.

8.1. Adrenergic crisis in phaeochromocytomas.

Mr J Clavijo.

Definition.
It is paroxysmal hypertension (> 140/90 mmHg) secondary to catecholamines released from a phaeochromocytoma and the consequential symptoms.

Aetiology.
Phaeochromocytomas are neuroendocrine tumours of the adrenal medulla. They may have extra-adrenal locations (paragangliomas, Zuckerkandl). They produce catecholamines, adrenaline being the most frequent. Catecholamines enter the venous blood via intra-abdominal hypertension (cough, sneeze, etc.) or spontaneously. They then lead to severe hypertension of varying duration. 90% are benign.

Diagnosis.
1. History: headaches, nervousness, flushing, sweating, irritability. Background: atypical or poorly controlled hypertension. Medications: antihypertensives.

2. Physical examination: BP, complications (CVA, cardiac ischaemia).

3. Investigations:
Blood: kidney and liver function. Full blood count.

Image: contrast-enhanced CT (Fig. 8.1) or MRI (elective).

Other: metanephrines in urine are diagnostic, with high sensitivity and specificity (elective).

Phaeochromocytoma complications:
- Multisystem: multiple organ failure. Pyrexia > 40° C. Hypertension, rarely hypotension.
- Cardiovascular: hypertensive crisis triggered by efforts, medications or anaesthesia. Cardiac failure, arrhythmias, cardiomyopathy, AAA, PVD, DVT.

- Respiratory: pulmonary oedema.
- Abdominal: digestive bleeding, ileus, perforated ulcer, mesenteric ischaemia.
- Neurologic: hemiplegia, seizures.
- Renal: ARF, haematuria.
- Metabolic: diabetic ketoacidosis. Lactic acidosis.

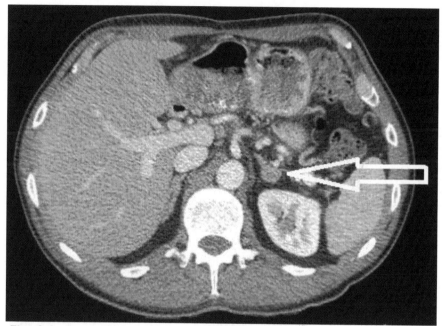

Fig. 8.1. Coronal view of CT. Arrow show uptake of left adrenal gland which is increased in size.

Treatment.
Medical.
Normalize blood pressure immediately. Most commonly used agents are Nifedipine and Nitrates. Nifedipine must be immediate release; bite and swallow is the best way to administer (not sublingual). Once the patient is stable, start pre-operative medical treatment, to prevent further crisis and intraoperative complications. Use an alpha blocker (Doxazosin 4 mg od), after 5 days add a beta blocker (Atenolol 50-100 mg od).

Surgical.
Curative treatment is done electively by adrenalectomy or resection of other catecholamine producing tissue. This can be done

laparoscopic by experienced urologists.

Complications.
Complications are the consequence of severe peripheral hypertension and include retinal and/or cerebral haemorrhage, myocardial infarction and seizures.

Outcomes.
If the elective (or rarely emergency) operation achieves the complete removal of all abnormal chromaffin tissue, blood pressure will return to normal.

Additional reading:
1. Diabetic and endocrine emergencies. Kearney T, Dang C. Postgrad Med J. 2007 Feb; 83(976): 79-86.
2. Undiagnosed phaeochromocytoma: the anesthesiologist nightmare. Myklejord DJ. Clin Med Res. 2004 Feb; 2(1): 59-62.
3. Phaeochromocytoma: a catecholamine and oxidative stress disorder. Pacak K. Endocr Regul. 2011 Apr; 45(2): 65-90.
4. Phaeochromocytoma. Foo M, Burton BJ, Ahmed R. Br J Hosp Med. 1995 Oct 4-17; 54(7): 318-21.
5. Hypertensive emergency due to phaeochromocytoma crisis complicated with refractory hemodynamic collapse. Hayıroğlu Mİ, Yıldırımtürk Ö, Bozbay M, Eren M, Pehlivanoğlu S. Turk Kardiyol Dern Ars. 2015 Dec; 43(8): 727-9.
6. Emergency resection of an extra-adrenal phaeochromocytoma: wrong or right? A case report and a review of literature. Bos JC, Toorians AW, van Mourik JC, van Schijndel RJ. Neth J Med. 2003 Aug; 61(8): 258-65.

8.2. Autonomic dysreflexia.

Mr J Clavijo and Mr T Rosenbaum.

Definition.

Autonomic dysreflexia (AD) is a massive unregulated autonomic sympathetic reflex response in patients with spinal cord injury (SCI) above the sympathetic level (T5-T6).

It is a rare but dangerous medical emergency characterised by a sudden elevation in blood pressure which requires immediate action. Clinician alertness is essential as SCI patients usually have no sensation or pain below the spinal cord level lesion.

Aetiology.

The nerve supply of the viscera is the autonomic nervous system which emerges from the brain stem and spinal cord at higher levels than the corresponding somatic nerves. All autonomic activity becomes disconnected from the somatic activity below the level of the cord injury.

A sensory input (generally not perceived due to the neurological lesion) usually from bladder or bowel, produces in the spinal cord a reflex with the output being a segmental sympathetic release. This leads to peripheral vasoconstriction and consequent hypertension. The baroreceptors in the carotid arteries detect the hypertension. The brain reacts by reducing the heart rate through the parasympathetic system (as far down as it can go due to the SCI). This bradycardia is insufficient to lower the blood pressure, and the hypertension continues. The sympathetic autonomic response prevails below the level of SCI, and the parasympathetic autonomic response prevails above it.

Frequency is 48-90% of all individuals who are injured at T6 and above. AD occurs during labour in approximately two thirds of pregnant women with SCI above the level of T6. Very careful monitoring and treatment is therefore clearly mandatory.

Diagnosis.

The diagnosis is clinical.

1. History: any stimulus below the level of the spinal injury can cause an episode of AD (pain and other sensations are obviously abolished below that level). Fig. 8.2.

Possible triggers to look for:
- Bladder distention
- Urinary tract infection
- Cystoscopy
- Urodynamics
- Detrusor-sphincter dyssynergia
- Epididymitis or scrotal compression
- Bowel distention
- Bowel impaction
- Gallstones
- Gastric ulcers or gastritis
- Invasive testing
- Haemorrhoids
- Gastro-colic irritation
- Appendicitis or other abdominal pathology
- Menstruation
- Pregnancy (especially labour and delivery)
- Vaginitis
- Sexual intercourse
- Ejaculation
- Deep vein thrombosis
- Pulmonary emboli
- Pressure ulcers
- Ingrown toenail
- Burns or sunburn
- Blisters
- Insect bites
- Contact with hard or sharp objects
- Temperature fluctuations
- Constrictive clothing, shoes, or appliances
- Fractures or other trauma
- Surgical or diagnostic procedures
- Pain (if some nociceptive sensation is preserved)

Symptoms:
a) Profuse sweating, especially in the face, neck, and shoulders.
b) Goose bumps.
c) Flushing of the skin especially in the face, neck, and shoulders;

this is a frequent symptom.
d) Blurred vision and spots in the visual field.
e) Nasal congestion, a common symptom.

Past medical history: previous episodes of AD. Ongoing medical problems.

2. Physical examination: sudden, significant rise in systolic and diastolic blood pressure.

Signs:
a) Abdomen: look for bladder distension, abdominal distension, pressure ulcers, and signs of acute abdomen.
b) PR for bowel impaction and haemorrhoids.
c) External genitalia: epididymitis, scrotal compression, turbid or offensive urine suggestive of urinary tract infection.
d) PV: menstruation, pregnancy, vaginitis.
e) Legs: deep vein thrombosis, pressure ulcers, ingrown toenail.
f) Generally: burns or sunburn, blisters, insect bites, fractures or other trauma. Profuse sweating above the level of lesion, especially in the face, neck, and shoulders; rarely occurs below the level of the lesion. Goose bumps above, or rarely below, the level of the lesion. Flushing of the skin above the level of the lesion, especially in the face, neck, and shoulders; this is a frequent sign.

3. Investigations:
Blood: routines including cultures and pregnancy test. FBC for infections.

Urine: dip and cultures (urinary tract infection).

Imaging: ultrasound scan may show bladder distension, gallstones, deep vein thrombosis. X rays and CT scan if fractures or other trauma are suspected.

If information is available from previous urodynamic studies: presence of detrusor-sphincter dyssynergia.

AUTONOMIC DYSREFLEXIA

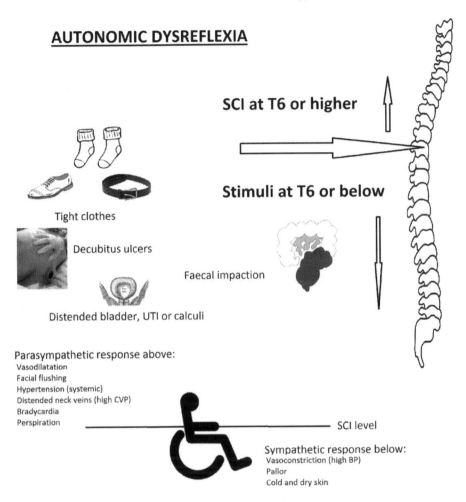

SCI at T6 or higher

Stimuli at T6 or below

Tight clothes

Decubitus ulcers

Faecal impaction

Distended bladder, UTI or calculi

Parasympathetic response above:
Vasodilatation
Facial flushing
Hypertension (systemic)
Distended neck veins (high CVP)
Bradycardia
Perspiration

SCI level

Sympathetic response below:
Vasoconstriction (high BP)
Pallor
Cold and dry skin

Fig. 8.2. Autonomic dysreflexia trigger stimuli.

Treatment.
Medical.
Sit up the patient immediately and loosen any clothing or constrictive devices. Sitting leads to pooling of blood in the lower extremities and may reduce blood pressure.

If an indwelling urinary catheter is not in place, catheterize the patient. If the patient has an indwelling urinary catheter, check the system along its entire length for kinks, folds, constrictions, obstructions and for correct placement.

Use an antihypertensive agent with rapid onset and short duration while the causes of AD are being investigated if the blood pressure is at or above 150 mm Hg systolic. The most commonly used agents are Nifedipine and nitrates (e.g., Nitroglycerine). Nifedipine should be in the immediate release form; bite and swallow is the preferred method of administering the drug, not sublingual administration.

Patients who have previously experienced episodes of AD are treated with antihypertensives prior to procedures known to cause this reaction.

Surgical treatment is necessary if there are trigger factors that require it for resolution.

Complications.
Complications associated with autonomic dysreflexia result from severe peripheral hypertension and include retinal and/or cerebral haemorrhage, myocardial infarction, seizures and death.

Outcomes.
Once the initial stimulus is removed, the hypertension resolves.

Additional reading:
1. The importance of autonomic dysreflexia to the urologist. Shergill IS, Arya M, Hamid R, Khastgir J, Patel HR, Shah PJ. BJU Int. 2004 May; 93(7): 923-6.
2. Autonomic dysreflexia and its urological implications: a review. Trop CS, Bennett CJ. J Urol. 1991 Dec; 146(6): 1461-9.
3. Autonomic dysreflexia: an important cardiovascular complication in spinal cord injury patients. Gunduz H, Binak DF. Cardiol J. 2012; 19(2): 215-9.
4. Autonomic dysreflexia: a medical emergency. Bycroft J, Shergill IS, Chung EA, Arya N, Shah PJ. Postgrad Med J. 2005 Apr; 81(954): 232-5.
5. Rehabilitation medicine: 1. Autonomic dysreflexia. Blackmer J. CMAJ. 2003 Oct 28; 169(9):931-5.

CHAPTER 9. Uro-Oncology Emergencies.

Mr J Clavijo.

We need to know oncological emergencies in Urology because most of the patients presenting with them are somehow under our care and usually under shared teams' care. All the conditions in this chapter do not necessarily belong in a Urology Syllabus, but the Urology team members need to be acutely aware of them, start adequate management and promptly refer the patient to our Oncology colleagues.

BCG complications are sometimes infectious, so the Bacteriology team helps enormously.

Metastatic SCC is oftentimes foreseeable and will require oncological and/or neurosurgical input. It can present as an AUR.

Hypercalcaemia has nothing to do with Urology; however, these patients can present with non-specific symptoms in the postoperative period of a debulking nephrectomy, and lead us to think of a surgical complication when the situation requires an equally urgent medical intervention.

Neutropenia in patients with urological conditions can present as a complicated UTI with an unusual clinical scenario and rapid progression.

Radiation cystitis is a debilitating collateral undesirable side effect. It requires a urological solution that has to consider quality of life and be proportionate to the symptoms.

9.1. Metastatic spinal cord compression in Urology.

Dr S Dixit and Mr J Clavijo.

Definition.
Neurological symptoms and signs caused by pressure over the spinal cord from the epidural extension of metastatic deposits in the vertebrae or from the paravertebral region. Similar features occurring at the vertebral level below L1, which is at or below the conus medullaris, is called cauda equina compression. Here forth discussion related to MSCC also applies to cauda equina compression, unless specified.

Prevalence.
5-10% of patients with cancer develop MSCC during the course of their disease. The risk increases to 28% in prostate cancer and 13% in renal cancer patients having bone metastases.

In prostate cancer, over one year, 10% of asymptomatic metastases in the vertebrae progress to clinical MSCC. This risk increased to 25% in 18 months and to 37% in 2 years in patients with castration resistant prostate cancer. The more significant risk factor is a PSA doubling time less than 3 months.

Aetiology.
1. Direct extension of the tumour from the vertebrae to the epidural space causing venous congestion, oedema, and venous ischemia. This is the most common pattern in patients with prostate cancer having sclerotic metastases. The onset is sub-acute with prodromal signs of worsening, localized or radicular pain, and leg weakness (Fig. 9.1).

2. Collapse or fracture of the vertebrae causing direct compression of the cord by the tumour or bone fragment. This type of MSCC is frequent with lytic metastases, more commonly observed with kidney cancer and bladder cancer. Patients with prostate cancer may also develop collapse or fracture of the vertebral body after a prolonged exposure to anti androgens and steroids.

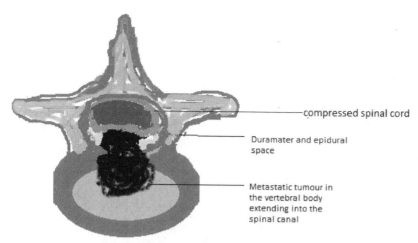

Fig. 9.1. Metastasis in the vertebral body extending into the spinal canal causing pressure over the dura mater and spinal cord.

The presentation of this type of MSCC is acute and warrants urgent intervention including steroids, spine stability measures, and neurosurgical intervention (Fig. 9.2).

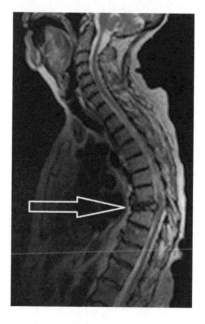

Fig. 9.2. MCC from a fracture of T8 vertebra (arrow).

3. Metastases at the para-spinal region can directly invade the epidural space through the intervertebral foramina. This type of presentation is rare in patients with urological cancer; however, it could arise from metastases in the ribs located at its origin near

the vertebral body, para-spinal soft issue metastases from kidney cancer, and para-aortic lymph node metastases from kidney and germ cell tumours. The onset of this type of compression is slow with the main presenting symptom being local and radicular pain (Fig. 9.3).

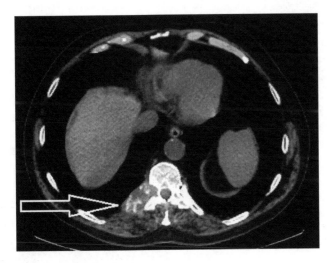

Fig. 9.3. Metastasis to the rib from renal cell cancer invading the spinal column (arrow).

4. Meningeal metastases: metastases to the leptomeninges in the subdural compartment are rare in urological cancer. Patients with kidney cancer may also have brain metastases and patients with prostate cancer usually have super scans with a very high PSA. Neurological symptoms and sings may indicate compression of the cord at multiple levels. Diagnosis is made through CSF cytology (lumbar puncture should be avoided in patients with hydrocephalus, multiple brain metastases, and in patients receiving anticoagulant and antiplatelet medication). Due to a high false negative rate of CSF cytology, Gadolinium contrast enhanced MRI is more useful in diagnosing meningeal metastases.

Diagnosis.
1. History: have a high risk of suspicion in patients with known vertebral metastases. Localized and radicular pain is the most common initial presenting feature. Patients often comment about tightness in the chest and pain radiating from back to the front for thoracic vertebral metastases and pain radiating down the leg in lumbar vertebral metastases. Patients may ignore the early sign of leg weakness and may attribute it to general weakness. It

is prudent to explore the history of leg weakness in detail by asking what patients cannot do now which they could do before. Often comments are 'my legs feel heavy, I feel wobbly, I feel my legs do not belong to me, and my legs cannot support me'. These comments warrant detailed neurological examination. If other causes are ruled out, as mentioned below in the differential diagnosis section, then there should be a lower threshold for arranging an MRI.

2. Neurological examination: elicit reflexes, assess the tone and power, establish any sensory level, and explore bladder and bowel sphincter functions. In the slowly developing MSCC (types 1 and 3 mentioned above), hyperreflexia and plantars going upwards are highly suggestive of MSCC. Loss of anal reflex, weak anal sphincter tone and saddle distribution of sensory loss are suggestive of cauda equina compression. In patients with a sudden onset of MSCC (type 2 mentioned above), the patients may present with spinal shock leading to hypotension, motor deficit, and loss of reflexes. Diminished sensory level below the dermatome involved in MSCC is more obvious in this type of presentation. Bladder and bowel motility dysfunction: MSCC above L2 level will lead to loss of voluntary bladder control but reflex emptying is maintained leading to frequency and urge incontinence. Cauda equina compression below L2 leads to retention and overflow incontinence.

3. Investigations.
Suspected direct extension of the tumour from the vertebrae to the epidural space = immediate x-ray of the vertebrae and an MRI within a week. Patients with prostate cancer having limited bone metastases (a small area of hotspot on a recent bone scan) which is responding to treatment, presenting with only localized pain or radiating pain but with normal reflexes and without any neurological symptoms or signs, may have an x-ray of the involved vertebral level to assess integrity. Arrange an MRI within a weeks' time.

Suspected collapse or fracture of the vertebrae causing direct compression of the cord: whole spine MRI should be done within 24 hrs. Particularly if the pain gets worse with coughing, radiates along the chest or down in the leg with the recent bone scan showing whole of the vertebral body involvement or extensive multiple spine metastases, but no neurological sings. The patients would need admission to monitor progression.

Suspected metastases at the para-spinal region: early MRI with monitoring following hospital admission would also be recommended in patients having previous bone scan (up to 6 months old) with recent progression of the disease or new presentation of prostate cancer with symptoms and signs as in previous cases, but no neurological signs.

An urgent whole spine MRI, immobilization, flat nursing with log-roll shifting should be arranged in patients presenting with radiating pain having either of these neurological signs and symptoms: plantar extension, hyper-reflexia, saddle anaesthesia with incontinence, and sudden severe spine pain. High dose Dexamethasone should be administered straight away. The MRI protocol involves T1- and T2-weighted images in axial, sagittal, and coronal plane. If MRI is contraindicated (patients with metallic cardiac valve or pacemaker), a CT scan is helpful.

Differential diagnosis (these conditions may co-exist with MSCC):
   A. Steroid induced proximal myopathy
   B. Sciatica
   C. Brain metastases
   D. Spondylolisthesis
   E. Osteoporotic fracture of a vertebra causing SCC

Patients with steroid induced proximal myopathy may present with the leg weakness. Absence of vertebral body tenderness and normal plantars and other reflexes would rule out MSCC. Weakness would be limited to thigh, gluteal, and shoulder muscles. Patients with brain metastases may have confusion. Weakness is usually more pronounced on one side. Clinically, sciatica, spondylolisthesis and osteoporotic fracture are difficult to differentiate from MSCC. MRI spine is useful in making a diagnosis. Diffusion-weighted imaging may be helpful in distinguishing between benign and pathologic compression fractures.

Treatment.
Medical.
1. Steroids. Immediate start of Dexamethasone. Give stat

intravenous 16 mg. Then 4 mg TDS or 8 mg BD orally or intravenously with proton pump inhibitors. Once a treatment for MSCC has been delivered, taper down Dexamethasone slowly by halving the dose every 3 to 6 days. An exposure to steroid over an extended period increases the risk of infections including fungal ones. Closely monitor blood sugar, mainly in known diabetics.

2. Immobilization. Immobilize the patient until plain x-ray or MRI rule out fracture or collapse of the spine. Collar should be used with cervical spine suspected MSCC. While transferring for imaging or for nursing, use pat slide and log-roll techniques. Resume mobility gradually after the completion of the treatment.

3. Radiotherapy. Every cancer centre should have a metastatic cord compression coordinator located at the centre delivering radiotherapy. Contact the coordinator or radiotherapy unit urgently, as soon as the MSCC is confirmed by an MRI or earlier if clinical presentation is very likely to be of MSCC.

4. Indications for radiotherapy:
   - Radiosensitive tumours such as prostate cancer, multiple myeloma, germ cell tumour, and lymphoma.
   - Following surgery.
   - Multiple level of cord compression.
   - Not fit for neurosurgical intervention.

Radiotherapy is given in 5 (20 Gy) or 10 (30 Gy) sessions (fractions) over one to two weeks. In patients with poor performance status and long standing established paraplegia a single session of 8 Gy is given for pain control. Temporary radiotherapy related side effects are diarrhoea, nausea (for lumbar area radiotherapy), sore throat, painful swallowing, and nausea (for thoracic and cervical area radiotherapy). These symptoms last for 1-3 weeks and respond to symptomatic medications.

5. Physiotherapy. Passive and then active physiotherapy is an integral part of the management to have long term improvement following surgery or radiotherapy. Patients should be encouraged to continue active physiotherapy on discharge at home.

6. Palliative care only. Treatment is not always necessary, and, in

some instances, may cause more discomfort. The patients with advanced disease, established paraplegia for many days, and limited life expectancy may get better palliative benefit by providing best supportive care. These patients should be spared the distress of transferring to a radiotherapy centre/unit and its related side effects. Various modelling scores have been developed to estimate the life expectancy of patients with MSCC and to identify the patients who may benefit with best supportive care only (without radiotherapy, surgery, aggressive steroid management, and active physiotherapy). The best supportive care includes a short course of steroid, passive physiotherapy, pain and other symptoms control, and defining an on-going care plan.

The patients with the following features could be managed with best supportive care:
- Performance status 4 before developing MSCC.
- Extensive visceral and bone metastases.
- Non-ambulatory with power zero on both legs for more than 7 days.

Surgery.
Contact Neurosurgeon on call urgently if decompression may be indicated.

Indications for spinal surgery:
- No diagnosis of primary.
- Vertebral body collapse or fracture.
- Life expectancy more than 3 months.
- Uncontrolled pain due to spine instability.
- MSCC limited to not more than one vertebral level.
- Medically fit to undergo a surgical intervention.
- Progression following radiotherapy.
- Radiotherapy resistant tumours such as kidney cancer.

Surgery involves decompression of the vertebral column by resection of the tumour and fixation of the adjacent vertebral bodies with pedicle screws and rods.

Outcomes.
1. Survival: patients with MSCC usually have poorer survival due to

associated advance metastatic disease in most of the patients and complications following MSCC. Patients who do not regain mobility are prone to have recurrent urinary and chest infections.

2. Recovery of mobility: recovery in gaining mobility or maintaining mobility is rather quick after surgery. Following radiotherapy, recovery starts in 1-2 weeks' time. The probability of recovery is 80% with hormone responsive disease, and if surgery or radiotherapy is carried out within 48 hours of developing leg weakness. The probability of re-gaining mobility decreases to only 20% if the treatment with surgery or radiotherapy is delayed more than 48 hours of onset of leg weakness. Patients with prostate cancer have a better outcome with radiotherapy compared to patients with renal cell cancer.

3. Recurrence: recurrence of MSCC at the same site is not uncommon. The risk of MSCC at other vertebral level depends on the extent of metastases, and the response of the disease to treatment. Multiple vertebral metastases, PSA doubling time less than 3 months and non-responding disease have a higher chance of recurrence of MSCC.

4. Prevention:
a) Increase awareness: educate patients with vertebral column metastases about the risk and complications of MSCC. Advise patients to contact their general practitioner immediately or attend accident & emergency/casualty if they start getting any of these symptoms:
   • A band like pain across the chest or abdomen associated with numbness in the legs.
   • Sudden onset or rapid deterioration of leg weakness leading to difficulty in walking.
   • Sudden onset of feeling of numbness over the gluteal area.
   • Sudden or rapid development of urine retention with overflow incontinence.

b) Bisphosphonates: Zoledronic acid 4mg given intravenously over 15 minutes in a saline drip repeated every 3 weeks has been shown to delay the occurrence of cord compression and fracture. In patients with hormone refractory and bone metastatic cancer, the risk of MSCC risk was reduced from 6.9 to 4.3% (not significant) over a follow up of 15 months. The dose should be reduced with decreasing GFR. Indication: multiple vertebral metastases with or without pain.

Toxicity of Zoledronic acid:

- Decreased renal function: monitor serum creatinine at every visit; reduce dose with lower GFR. Contraindicated if dehydrated and GFR less than 40ml/minute.
- Jaw necrosis: the risk of mandibular and maxillary necrosis is 1.4%. To reduce the risk the patients should have a dentist opinion before starting Zoledronic acid. Dental extraction or any dental invasive procedure should be done before starting and should be avoided if patients are on Zoledronic acid. If any dental invasive procedure is mandatory, it should be stopped for at least 3-4 weeks. Encourage the patients to use regular mouthwash and maintain good oral hygiene.
- Hypocalcaemia: monitor serum calcium and supplement oral calcium/vitamin D tablets.
- Temporary flu like symptoms are managed with paracetamol.

c) Denosumab: is a monoclonal antibody, which inhibits osteoclasts by binding receptor activator of nuclear factor-κB (RANK). Denosumab is given 120mg subcutaneously every 4 weeks to prevent skeletal related events in castrate resistant metastatic prostate cancer. It has shown similar efficacy to Zoledronic acid in delaying MSCC in patients with castrate resistant metastatic prostate cancer. After a median exposure of 10-11 months, the risk of MSCC was 3% with Denosumab compared to 4% with Zoledronic acid. However, the median time to onset of any first skeletal related events, including fracture, need of radiotherapy, and MSCC, was significantly longer with Denosumab (20.7 months vs.17 months).

d) The risk of jaw necrosis is 2% and hypocalcaemia 13% compared with 1% and 6% respectively with Zoledronic acid. Denosumab does not affect renal function. Given 60mg subcutaneously every 6 months decreased three year cumulative incidence of vertebral fracture in hormone sensitive non-metastatic prostate cancer from 3.9 % to 1.5% (statistically significant).

e) Vertebroplasty of collapsed vertebra: image guided injection of bone cement into the collapsed vertebral body helps in relieving pain and provides spine stability. However, presently there is no evidence that vertebroplasty reduces the risk of MSCC. This procedure is not indicated in patients with impending or established MSCC.

f) Life style: patients with spine metastases should avoid lifting heavy weights and movements which involve twisting the spine. Non-weight-bearing muscle strengthening resistance exercises should be recommended.

g) Screening with MRI: presently there is no evidence of screening for or monitoring the development of MSCC from known bony vertebral metastases. It would be prudent to have a base line MRI in high-risk patients having extensive vertebral metastases on bone scan or fast rising PSA with doubling time of less than 3 months.

h) Communication with the patients and their family members: keep patients and their family members (after permission from the patients) informed about the cause, severity, the treatment options, and prognosis of the cord compression. Often, patients have unrealistic expectations of recovery. Incomplete or lack of recovery leads to disappointment and frustration leading to un-satisfaction and loss of confidence in the treating team. Timely and realistic outcomes information helps patients to plan their future commitments, life events, life style, and provide an opportunity to plan ahead their day-to day activities.

Register all the discussions with the patients and other medical professionals. Keep annotation up-to-date about progress in management.

Additional reading:

1. Spinal Surgery for Palliation in Malignant Spinal Cord Compression. Akram, H. and J. Allibone. Clinical oncology. 22(9): 792-800. 2010.
2. Spinal Cord compression. Baehring, J. In: DeVita, Hellman, and Rosenberg's Cancer Principles & Practice of Oncology. J. V. De Vita, Lawrence TS, Rosenberg SA. Philadelphia, Lippincott Williams & Wilkins. 2: 2441. 2008.
3. Early diagnosis and treatment is crucial for neurological recovery after surgery for metastatic spinal cord compression in prostate cancer. Crnalic, S., C. Hildingsson, et al. Acta Oncol. 2012.
4. An extended role for CT in the emergency diagnosis of malignant spinal cord compression. Crocker, M., R. Anthantharanjit, et al. Clinical radiology 66(10): 922-927. 2011.

5. Denosumab versus Zoledronic acid for treatment of bone metastases in men with castration-resistant prostate cancer: a randomised, double-blind study. Fizazi, K., M. Carducci, et al. Lancet 377(9768): 813-822. 2011.

6. Acute morbidity reduction using 3DCRT for prostate carcinoma: a randomized study. Koper, P. C. M., J. C. Stroom, et al. International journal of radiation oncology, biology, physics 43(4): 727-734. 1999.

7. Hemorrhagic cystitis following radiotherapy for stage Ib cancer of the cervix. Levenback, C., P. J. Eifel, et al. Gynecol Oncol 55(2): 206-210. 1994.

8. Sensitivity and specificity of MRI in detecting malignant spinal cord compression and in distinguishing malignant from benign compression fractures of vertebrae. Li, K. C. and P. Y. Poon. Magn Reson Imaging 6(5): 547-556. 1988.

9. Skeletal complications in patients with bone metastases from renal cell carcinoma and therapeutic benefits of Zoledronic acid. Lipton, A., A. Colombo-Berra, et al. Clin Cancer Res 10(18 Pt 2): 6397S-6403S. 2004.

10. Zoledronic Acid Is Superior to Pamidronate in the Treatment of Hypercalcemia of Malignancy: A Pooled Analysis of Two Randomized, Controlled Clinical Trials. Major, P., A. Lortholary, et al. Journal of Clinical Oncology 19(2): 558-567. 2001.

11. Metastatic spinal cord compression guidance. NICE. 2008.

12. Bone metastases from solid tumours - Denosumab: guidance. NICE. 2012

13. Pathologic fracture and metastatic spinal cord compression in patients with prostate cancer and bone metastases. Nieder, C., E. Haukland, et al. BMC Urol 10: 23. 2010.

14. A Randomized, Placebo-Controlled Trial of Zoledronic Acid in Patients With Hormone-Refractory Metastatic Prostate Carcinoma. Saad, F., D. M. Gleason, et al. Journal of the National Cancer Institute 94(19): 1458-1468. 2002.

15. Zoledronic acid is effective in preventing and delaying skeletal events in patients with bone metastases secondary to genitourinary cancers. Saad, F. and A. Lipton BJU Int 96(7): 964-969. 2005.

16. Denosumab in men receiving androgen-deprivation therapy for prostate cancer. Smith, M. R., B. Egerdie, et al. N Engl J Med 361(8): 745-755. 2009.

17. Frequency of screening magnetic resonance imaging to detect occult spinal cord compromise and to prevent neurological deficit in metastatic castration-resistant prostate cancer. Venkitaraman, R., S. A. Sohaib, et al. Clin Oncol (R Coll Radiol) 22(2): 147-152. 2010.

18. Skeletal complications and survival in renal cancer patients with bone metastases. Woodward, E., S. Jagdev, et al. Bone 48(1): 160-166. 2011.

9.2. Intravesical BCG treatment complications.

Mr J Clavijo.

Definition.
Intravesical administration of Bacillus Calmette-Guerin (BCG), a live attenuated strain of Mycobacterium bovis, has become a mainstay of adjunctive therapy for superficial bladder cancer. There are several strains of BCG, but none has proved more effective than others, the same applies to the number of colony forming units (CFU) used. The description of the technique is beyond the scope of this chapter.

Intravesical BCG treatment indications: patients who have superficial (NMIBC), CIS or grade 3 (high grade) bladder transitional cell carcinomas and selected grade 2. Early recurrence post TURBT.

For pTa-pT1 grade 2, intravesical Mitomycin is practically equally effective and has considerable less adverse effects.

Intravesical BCG treatment contraindications:
- Urinary tract infections.
- Haematuria.
- Patients who had transurethral resection or biopsy in the last 4 weeks.
- Traumatic bladder catheterization in the preceding week.
- Active tuberculosis.
- Anti-tuberculosis drugs (Streptomycin, PAS, Isoniazid, Rifampicin, Ethambutol). Ongoing TB treatment.
- Immune deficiency: congenital, acquired, iatrogenic, drugs or other therapies.
- HIV positive.
- Pregnancy, lactation.
- Fever.
- Bladder radiotherapy.

Classification.
Systemic (<1%) and vesical (5%) complications. In general, 95% of the patients have no serious side effects.

Bladder side effects.
- About 2 out of 3 people have cystitis and dysuria.
- About 7 out of 10 people have frequency.
- About 1 in 4 people have haematuria.
- About 1 in 2 people have flu like symptoms for 24 to 48 hours after each treatment (such as fever, chills, and fatigue -asthenia).
- About 1 or 2 out of 100 people have arthralgia (painful joints).

Evaluation.: MSU to rule out bacterial infection, CXR.

Treatment.
Options vary according to the severity of toxicity from delaying to withholding instillations. Perform symptomatic management of flu like symptoms. Increase diuresis for haematuria or start bladder irrigation if needed. Use anticholinergics for frequency. Some patients find relief from Cranberry products.

Systemic side effects.
Rarely, BCG can spread through the body, leading to a life-threatening infection. Systemic side effects vary from mild malaise and fever to, in rare instances, life-threatening or fatal sepsis.

Systemic BCG symptoms:
- Fever and chills.
- Arthralgia (joint pain).
- Feeling sick or vomiting.
- Cough.
- Dermatitis (skin rash).
- Asthenia.
- Confusion or dizziness.

Adverse effects on the genitourinary tract: symptomatic granulomatous prostatitis, orchitis, ureter obstruction, urethral strictures or renal abscess.

Evaluation: MSU to rule out bacterial infection, CXR. Blood culture for TB.

Treatment.

When disseminated BCG infection occurs, withhold instillations. Anti-tuberculous therapy (Isoniazid and Rifampicin) with or without glucocorticoids should be administered for up to 6 months.

Despite its toxicity, the risk-benefit ratio favours the use of BCG in patients who have high-risk tumours and it is an option for intermediate ones in non-muscle invasive bladder transitional cell carcinoma.

Additional reading:

1. BCG intravesical instillations: recommendations for side-effects management. Rischmann P, Desgrandchamps F, Malavaud B, Chopin DK. Eur Urol. 2000; 37 Suppl 1:33-6.
2. Complications of intravesical BCG immunotherapy. Uptodate. http://www.uptodate.com/contents/complications-of-intravesical-bcg-immunotherapy?source=search_result&search=complications+ofintravesical+bcg+immunotherapy&selectedTitle=1~150. On 04/04/2016.
3. Bladder cancer treatment. Treatment into the bladder. Cancer Research UK. http://www.cancerresearchuk.org/about-cancer/type/bladder-cancer/treatment/early/treatment-into-the-bladder. On 08/04/2016.
4. Incidence and treatment of complications of bacillus Calmette-Guerin intravesical therapy in superficial bladder cancer. Lamm DL, van der Meijden PM, Morales A, Brosman SA, Catalona WJ, Herr HW, Soloway MS, Steg A, Debruyne FM. J Urol. 1992 Mar; 147(3): 596-600.
5. Marker tumour response to Evans and Pasteur bacille Calmette-Guérin in multiple recurrent pTa/pT1 bladder tumours: report from the Medical Research Council Subgroup on Superficial Bladder Cancer (Urological Cancer Working Party). Fellows GJ, Parmar MK, Grigor KM, Hall RR, Heal MR, Wallace DM. Br J Urol. 1994 Jun; 73(6): 639-44.

9.3. Hypercalcaemia from Urology malignancies.

Mr J Clavijo.

Definition.
It is serum calcium over 10.5 mg/dl or 2.6 mmol/L. Hypercalcaemia can cause arrhythmias, and an increase in the production of gastrin with consequent gastritis or gastric ulcers (including perforation).

Aetiology.
Metastases to the bone produce a release of calcium. The most frequent urology cancers involved are prostate cancer and renal cell cancer. In renal cancer and phaeochromocytoma there can also be PTH-like production that increases serum calcium, as a para-neoplastic syndrome. Calcium can also be elevated as a consequence of prolonged immobilization, renal failure and rhabdomyolysis.

High calcium reduces neuro-muscular excitability.

99% of body calcium is in the bones, and only 0.1% is extracellular (serum).

Classification.
- Mild: <12 mg/dl.
- Moderate: 12-14 mg/dl.
- Severe: >14 mg/dl.

Diagnosis.
1. History:
CNS: cognitive difficulties, anxiety, depression, confusion and coma.
Neuro-muscular system: fatigue or muscle weakness, myalgia.
Renal: polyuria and polydipsia, dehydration.
Gastrointestinal: nausea and vomiting, anorexia, constipation, abdominal pain, gastritis.
Skeletal: bone pain, osteoporosis.
Cardiovascular: hypertension, shortened QT interval, wide T wave, Osborn wave, cardiac arrhythmias.

Past medical history: urinary lithiasis, nephrocalcinosis, vascular calcification, myocardial hypertrophy. Presence of bone metastasis. Familial hypercalcaemia. Drug history: diuretics, anti-cancer drugs, hormonal treatment, vitamin D, lithium.

2.   Physical examination: mainly neuro-muscular. Tone and reflexes.

3.   Investigations:
Blood: U&E, Calcaemia, Mg, eventually PTH.

Imaging: when patient stable, KUB USS and KUB X-ray and bone scan.

Others: periodic ECGs or monitoring. Fig. 9.4.

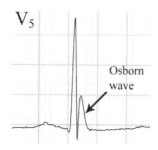

Fig. 9.4. ECG showing Osborn wave.

Treatment.
Medical.
First and foremost, are there advanced directives? The decision whether or not to treat hypercalcaemia (and how) when it is caused by cancer depends on the objectives of cancer treatment in general. Treatment of hypercalcaemia can reduce pain, improve quality of life, and allow the patient to resume activity and undergo specific treatments for their cancer.

Mild hypercalcaemia can be treated electively with bisphosphonates.

Moderate and severe cases: correcting calcium level is the priority. Do it by prompt rehydration. This usually needs to be done IV with saline. Resuscitate as needed. Severe hypercalcaemia (>14 mg/dL or 3.5 mmol/l) may need ITU monitoring, as fluid replacement may need to be done with CVP control and permanent cardiac monitoring. When stable, add Furosemide, 40 mg IV. If in renal failure, patient may need hemofiltration, particularly if diuresis is not recovered after initial hydration management.

Additionally act upon the hypercalcaemia source by adding Zoledronic acid, Denosumab or Calcitonin (which is fast acting) according to the local Oncology protocol.

Complications.
The more relevant complications of hypercalcaemia are coma and death.

Related to treatment: avoid pulmonary oedema when rehydrating the patient.

Outcomes.
Hypercalcaemia can usually be corrected. The presence of metastasis, however, gives a poor prognosis, especially in renal cancer.

Additional reading:
1. Clinical practice. Hypercalcaemia associated with cancer. Stewart AF. N Engl J Med. 2005 Jan 27; 352 (4): 373-9.
2. A Practical Approach to Hypercalcemia. Carroll MF, Schade DS. Am Fam Physician. 2003 May 1; 67(9):1959-1966.
3. BCCA Protocol Summary Guidelines for the Diagnosis and Management of Malignancy Related Hypercalcemia. British Columbia Cancer Agency. http://www.bccancer.bc.ca/chemotherapy-protocols-site/Documents/Supportive%20Care/SCHYPCAL_Protocol_1Oct2012_rev.pdf. On 08/04/2016.
4. Acute Hypercalcaemia: emergency endocrine guidance. Society for Endocrinology. https://www.endocrinology.org/policy/docs/13-02_EmergencyGuidance-AcuteHypercalcaemia.pdf. On 08/04/2016.

9.4. Radiation cystitis and proctitis.

Dr S Dixit and Mr J Clavijo.

A. Radiation Cystitis.

Definition.
Radiation cystitis is an adverse unintended and undesirable event occurring during and after the course of radiotherapy. The reaction of the bladder to radiation often presents with the cystitis syndrome which is similar to the infective aetiology.

Aetiology.
Radiation cystitis can occur following radiotherapy to any pelvic tumour with decreasing frequency observed with cancer of the cervix, uterus, prostate and the bladder. The risk of radiation cystitis increases with higher radiation dose, larger volume of the bladder and other co morbidities including diabetes, hypertension and other vascular disorders. Patients with prostate cancer with underlying urinary symptoms are at a greater risk of having acute radiation cystitis.

Incidence: with standard radiotherapy, 66 Gy to the prostate, with 3-D conformal radiotherapy: 47% grade 1, 17% grade 2 and 2% grade > 2 urological toxicity.

Classification.
Any radiation reaction is classified as acute or late. Acute radiation reaction occurs during or up to 3 months of completion of radiotherapy. Late reactions usually start 6 months following completion of radiotherapy.

Diagnosis and treatment.
1. Acute radiation cystitis.
These are unintended events (a complication) occurring during and up to 3 months following the course of radiotherapy. Mostly these are temporary and resolve with medical and conservative management. Signs and symptoms are similar to any infective cystitis and overactive bladder. Symptoms build up from the second week of

starting radiotherapy and peak 1-2 weeks later, before normalizing in 4-8 weeks' time. Symptoms are increased frequency, urgency, dysuria, urge incontinence and rarely, mainly in prostate cancer, retention.

Radiation Therapy Oncology Group (RTOG) criteria of grading acute radiation cystitis:

Grade 1	Grade 2	Grade 3	Grade 4
Frequency of urination or nocturia twice pre-treatment habit, dysuria, urgency not requiring medication	Frequency of urination or nocturia which is less frequent than every hour. Dysuria, urgency, bladder spasm requiring local anaesthetic (e.g., Phenazopyridine)	Frequency with urgency and nocturia hourly or more frequently; dysuria, pelvic pain or bladder spasm requiring regular or frequent narcotics; gross haematuria with or without clot passage	Haematuria requiring transfusion; acute bladder obstruction not secondary to clot passage; ulceration or necrosis

Management of acute radiation cystitis: it is important to explain patients that these are expected side effects which do need attention if they get worse.

- Grade 1: needs assurance, encourage to increase fluid intake, rule out infection, alkalinise urine with Potassium citrate (10ml in a cup of water to drink three or four times a day, watch for serum potassium, mainly in diabetics o renal failure). Cranberry juice has also been found useful in some patients. Radiation therapy could be continued.
- Grade 2: manage as grade 1 and add an anticholinergic such is such as Oxybutynin. Watch for retention in patients with prostate cancer. Radiation therapy could be continued.
- Grade 3: manage as grade 2, increase the dose of Oxybutynin, or choose another anticholinergic, use opioids such as Morphine or anti-inflammatories such Diclofenac. If it doesn't get better then patients need admission. Radiotherapy may be interrupted if symptoms don't get better.
- Grade 4: stop radiotherapy, needs an urgent admission, intravenous fluid, bladder irrigation, anticholinergic, opioids and

supportive measures.

2. Late radiation cystitis.

This usually starts 6 months after radiotherapy. The risk may continue to increase up to 3 years following radiotherapy. Symptoms are macroscopic haematuria, bladder contracture and low compliance, causing increased frequency and urgency, bladder ulcer(s) causing pelvic pain and dysuria. Pathologically new and abnormal capillary formation which in cystoscopy are seen as telangiectasia, endarteritis, fibrosis and mucosal ulcers.

Pathology: tissues undergo a progressive deterioration marked by a reduction of small blood vessels and fibrosis. These events may be exacerbated by infection or surgical involvement in the affected area. Moreover, the most damaging effects of radiotherapy are due to obliterative endarteritis. If present, haemorrhagic cystitis typically presents between 6 months and 10 years after radiotherapy.

Cystoscopy findings: on cystoscopy radiation injury is characterized by changes such as:
- Telangiectasia.
- Diffuse erythema.
- Prominent sub mucosal vascularity.
- Mucosal oedema.

Grading is according to standard criteria for adverse events (Clavien-Dindo):

Grade	Description
1	Microscopic haematuria; minimal increase in frequency, urgency, dysuria, or nocturia; new onset of incontinence
2	Moderate haematuria; moderate increase in frequency, urgency, dysuria, nocturia or incontinence; urinary catheter placement or bladder irrigation indicated; limiting some daily life activities
3	Gross haematuria; transfusion, IV medications or hospitalization indicated; elective endoscopic, radiologic or operative intervention indicated
4	Life-threatening consequences; urgent radiologic or operative intervention indicated
5	Death

Management of late radiation cystitis:

- Grade 1: needs cystoscopy, encourage fluid intake and empty bladder regularly, anticholinergics. Rule out other causes of cystitis (culture).

- Grade 2: cystoscopy, bladder irrigation, other management as for grade1.

- Grade 3: as grade 2 plus medical therapy: Pentoxyphylline, Oestrogens, hyperbaric oxygen. Local therapy: irrigation, cystoscopy and fulguration, local sclerotherapy, Formalin.

Pentoxyphylline has been shown to relieve pain due to radiation fibrosis. It improves the flow of blood by decreasing its viscosity. This increases blood flow to the affected microcirculation and enhances tissue oxygenation.

Oestrogen derivatives have been used to correct prolonged bleeding time. The mechanism of action of conjugated oestrogens in radiation cystitis is unknown. In patients with renal failure, oestrogen has been reported to correct prolonged bleeding time. However, in radiation cystitis complications, bleeding time is usually normal. Dose is Stilboestrol 5mg/day orally for 4-7 days. Conjugated oestrogens have a response rate of 100%, and the recurrence rate is 20%.

Hyperbaric oxygen (HBO): if significant fibrosis and ischemia have already occurred, HBO therapy does not reverse the changes and only prevents further injury. HBO therapy has a reported response rate of 27-92%, and the recurrence rate is 8-63%. It is administered as 100% oxygen at 2-2.5atm. Each session lasts from 90-120 minutes, and patients receive sessions 5 days weekly for a total of 40-60 sessions.

Local sclerotherapy: in selected patients intractable haematuria could be controlled with injection of a sclerosing agent (e.g., 1% Ethoxysclerol) into the haemorrhagic area on the bladder mucosa.

Bladder irrigation: in order of increasing toxicity, these agents include saline, 1% Alum, Aminocaproic acid solution, and 1-10% Formalin.
a) Formalin, a 37% solution of Formaldehyde and water

compounded at the pharmacy, is a tissue fixative. For bladder irrigation, a 1-10% solution (4% preferred) is used. Manually fill the bladder to capacity under gravity (solution bag < 15cm above the symphysis pubis to control pressure); contact time ranges from 14 minutes for a 10% solution to 23 minutes for a 5% solution. This is a painful procedure and requires a general anaesthetic. The response rate is 52-89%, and the recurrence rate is 20-25%.

b) Aminocaproic acid 2.5% solution (2.5 g in 100 cc of normal saline) for 1 hour, three times a day.

c) Alum, which is also compounded at the pharmacy, causes protein precipitation in the interstitial spaces and cell membranes, causing contraction of the extra cellular matrix and tamponade of bleeding vessels. Exposed capillary epithelium also scleroses. A 1% solution is prepared by mixing 50g of Potassium aluminium sulphate in 5L of distilled water; it is run intravesical at a rate of 3-5mL/min and increased to a maximum of 10mL/min if returns are not clear; it is continued for 6 hours after bleeding stops. Alum has a response rate of 50-80%, and the recurrence rate is 10%.

- Grade 3-4: additional surgical procedures include: percutaneous nephrostomy, internal iliac artery embolization, ileostomy, and cystectomy. All these are options if the bleeding persists, there is obstruction or symptoms become unresponsive to other approaches.

B. Radiation Proctitis.

Definition.
It is the inflammation and damage to the rectum after radiotherapy. Just like in radiation cystitis these are adverse unintended and undesirable events occurring during and after the course of treatment. Present in 8 to 14% of patients with pelvic radiotherapy.

Aetiology.
Post radiation ischaemic endarteritis. This can lead to fibrosis, angiodysplasia and ulcers. Almost 50% of patients with pelvic malignancies are candidates for radiation therapy at one point.

Classification.
Radiation injury can be divided into acute and chronic.

An acute injury occurs within six weeks of radiation treatment. Symptoms associated with acute radiation proctitis include diarrhoea, urgency, faecal incontinence, and rectal bleeding.

Chronic radiation proctitis happens in up to 75% of patients receiving pelvic radiation. May appear months to decades after treatment. Symptoms are similar to those experienced in an acute injury. It's a progressive disease.

Diagnosis.
1. History: diarrhoea, urgency, pain and tenesmus. Bleeding, fistulae and occlusion can also occur in severe cases.

Past medical history: radiotherapy protocol and previous digestive conditions. Drug history: past and present. Anticoagulation or antiplatelets.

2. Physical examination: rule out peritonitis. DRE can be painful, if in doubt, postpone it, do it under GA, and/or ask a colo-rectal surgeon to see the patient.
3. Investigations:
Blood: FBC, U&Es.

Imaging: CT if complications are suspected.

Others: arrange a colonoscopy, where diagnosis and disease extent can be confirmed. It can also allow treatment by Argon Beam Coagulation of abnormal areas.

Treatment.
Medical.
Acute: if symptoms persist and are mild, antidiarrheals may be enough to manage them. Balsalazide, Sulfasalazine, Mesalazine and Olsalazine can be used as liquid or foam enemas, or suppositories. Same applies to Hydrocortisone, Sucralfate and Amifostine.

Hyperbaric oxygen therapy can be used electively.

Surgical.
Only considered when everything else fails, as bowel anastomoses tend to dehisce in radiated patients. Surgical treatment is individualized based on the patient's condition and the intraoperative findings. Anastomotic breakdown is about 50% (with a grim prognosis).

Complications.
Fistulae and bowel occlusion.

Outcomes.
Surgical procedures on radiated bowel have morbidity rates of 12-65% and mortality rates of 2-13%. Almost 50% of patients who survive a laparotomy for radiation bowel injury require another operation for further bowel damage from radiation. In these, the mortality rate is 25%.

Additional reading:

1. Chemical- and radiation-induced haemorrhagic cystitis: current treatments and challenges. Payne H, Adamson A, Bahl A, Borwell J, Dodds D, Heath C, Huddart R, McMenemin R, Patel P, Peters JL, Thompson A. BJU Int. 2013. Nov; 112(7): 885-97.
2. The use of the hyperbaric oxygenation therapy in urology. Passavanti G. Arch Ital Urol Androl. 2010 Dec; 82(4):173-6.
3. Management of radiation cystitis. Smit SG, Heyns CF. Nat Rev Urol. 2010 Apr; 7(4):206-14.
4. Urologic emergencies in the cancer patient. Russo P. Semin Oncol. 2000 Jun; 27(3): 284-98.
5. Non-surgical interventions for late radiation proctitis in patients who have received radical radiotherapy to the pelvis. Denton A, Forbes A, Andreyev J, Maher EJ. Cochrane Database Syst Rev. 2002 ; (1): CD003455.
6. The management of intractable haematuria. Choong SK, Walkden M, Kirby R. BJU Int. 2000 Dec; 86(9): 951-9.
7. Intravesicular instillation of E-aminocaproic acid for patients with adenovirus-induced hemorrhagic cystitis. Lakhani A, Raptis A, Frame D, Simpson D, Berkahn L, Mellon-Reppen S, Klingemann H. Bone Marrow Transplant. 1999 Dec; 24(11): 1259-60.
8. Guidelines for the diagnosis, prevention and management of chemical- and radiation-induced cystitis. Payne H, Thompson A, Adamson A, Bahl A, Borwell J, Dodds D, Heath C, Peters J. Journal of Clinical Urology. 2014; 7 (1): 25-35.
9. Hemorrhagic cystitis: A challenge to the urologist. Manikandan R, Kumar S, Dorairajan LN. Indian Journal of Urology. 2010; 26(2): 159-166.

9.5. Neutropenic sepsis.

Mr J Clavijo.

Definition.

Neutropenia is an abnormally low level of neutrophils. The normal range is 2.5-7.5 x 10^9/L. Moderate neutropenia is 0.5-1.0 x 10^9/L. Severe neutropenia under 0.5 x 10^9/L. Some degree of neutropenia occurs in about half of people with cancer who are receiving chemotherapy. Neutropenia is the main predisposing factor of an infection in a patient with cancer. It's associated with substantial morbidity, mortality, and costs.

Aetiology.

Hematopoietic system suppression secondary to:
A. Chemotherapy.
B. Metastases to bone marrow.
C. Radiation therapy that affects the bone marrow.
D. Hemato-oncology conditions.

Elderly and frail patients with severe or long-lasting neutropenia are more likely to develop an infection. For patients with neutropenia, even a minor infection can quickly become systemic. Nadir count is about seven to 14 days after chemo.

Classification.

A. High risk: severe symptoms, hypotension, dehydration, age over 70.
B. Low risk: outpatient, mild symptoms, normotensive, well hydrated, age under 60.

Diagnosis.

1. History:
- Temperature, chills or sweating.
- Abdominal pain.
- Pain in the peri-anal area.
- Dysuria or frequent urination.
- Diarrhoea or sores around the anus.
- Inflammation around a wound, or the site of intravenous catheter insertion.
- Unusual vaginal discharge or itching.

Past medical history: tumour, treatment regime and when it happened. Drug history: past and present.

2. Physical examination: look for foci. Rule out UTI and peritonitis.

3. Investigations:
Blood: FBC, blood cultures from a peripheral vein, and any venous catheters. Blood film, D-dimer and fibrinogen to look for disseminated intravascular coagulation. U&E, LFTs, CRP, ESR, coagulation screen.

Imaging: CXR and CT.

Others: urine culture or other foci.

Treatment.
Medical.
Successful management depends on early recognition. Resuscitate and re-hydrate the patient. Better survival if managed by a multi-specialty team. Intravenous Piperacillin and Tazobactam. Aminoglycosides should not be used for initial empirical therapy, unless the focus is a clear UTI.

Chemotherapy dose reductions and delays, and colony-stimulating factors can be later initiated by the Oncology team.

Surgical.
Drain any foci found.

Complications.
5% of cases will need ITU.

Outcomes.
Overall mortality is approximately 5% to 11%. Mortality is 18% in Gram-negative and 5% in Gram-positive bacteraemia.

Additional reading:
1. Neutropenic sepsis: prevention and management in people with cancer. NICE Clinical Guideline. National Institute for Health and Care Excellence. https://www.nice.org.uk/guidance/cg151. On 08/04/2016.
2. Management of febrile neutropenia: ESMO Clinical Practice Guidelines. de Naurois J,

Novitzky-Basso I, Gill MJ, Marti FM, Cullen MH, Roila F; ESMO Guidelines
Working Group. Ann Oncol. 2010 May; 21 Suppl 5: 252-6.

3. Chemotherapy-induced neutropenia: risks, consequences, and new directions for its
management. Crawford J, Dale DC, Lyman GH. Cancer. 2004 Jan 15; 100(2): 228-37.

CHAPTER 10. Acute Pain Management in Urology.

Dr E Evans and Dr A Asumang.

Introduction.

Urological surgery is an area of medicine in which the management of pain can be problematic. The patients are often complex, with a variety of co-morbidities and pathologies that can make assessment and management of pain challenging. Patients may be suffering due to pre-existing problems (for example arthritis), their presenting urological problem (for example renal colic), or following surgical intervention (for example following nephrectomy). The management of pain can be further complicated by the potential for altered renal function, and by any comorbidity that require special consideration. As a doctor caring for patients with urological problems, a thorough understanding of the assessment and management of pain is crucial, to ensure that these patients are well managed and have the best possible experience and outcomes.

1. Why Pain Relief is Important?

Pain management is an important aspect of care for all patients. The reasons why good pain management is so vital are varied, and can be broadly divided into psychological and physiological factors.

Psychological: uncontrolled pain can undermine confidence in the surgical and nursing teams. Patients who experience ongoing pain are less likely to be willing to comply with treatments, potentially increasing length of stay in hospital. Pain also disturbs sleep, can worsen confusion and delirium, and can be extremely distressing to both patients and relatives. With persistent pain, some patients may develop psychological sequelae akin to post-traumatic stress disorder.

Physiological: pain increases heart rate and blood pressure, as a result of activation of the sympathetic nervous system. This results in an increase in oxygen consumption, and in susceptible patients, a higher risk of cardio-respiratory sequelae. Patients with poor pain control are also more likely to have poor mobility, which puts them at increased risk of complications, for example venous thromboembolism.

In short, good pain management reduces complications, decreases length of stay in hospital, and leads to a more positive patient experience. As many of the procedures involved in urological surgery can cause significant discomfort it is important that doctors caring for this group have a thorough understanding of how to assess and treat pain and some knowledge of the complications or side effects of the analgesia.

2. Assessment of pain.

Patients presenting with pain in the urology setting may be experiencing discomfort for a variety of different reasons. They may have chronic pain issues prior to admission, from an unrelated medical condition, or as a result of their urological problem. Alternatively the pain they experience could be acute, either due to the underlying pathology or because the patient has had surgery.

Whatever the cause of pain, the strategy to assess and treat should be the same. First, a thorough history should be taken. The aim of this is to establish the likely underlying cause of the pain, in order to inform management. This history should follow a structure to ensure nothing is missed. A suggested strategy is the SOCRATES mnemonic, which covers most important aspects of pain assessment. This stands for:

Site: the site of pain can give useful clues to the likely underlying cause.

Onset: when the pain started, and what the patient was doing at the time.

Character: how the pain feels- stabbing/burning/crushing, colicky etc.

Radiation: if the pain moves anywhere, such as to the groin.

Associated features: other symptoms associated with the pain, e.g. nausea and vomiting.

Time course: how long the pain lasts for and when it is at its worst.

Exacerbating/alleviating factors: what makes the pain better or worse. This can also include the effect of any analgesic medication already prescribed.

Severity: how bad the pain is.

Common urological presentations.

- Urolithiasis and renal colic: classically a severe pain which is localised to one side and radiates from "loin to groin", and is colicky in nature.
- Prostatic pain: multiple possible causes, including infection, malignancy and benign prostatic hypertrophy. Pain is usually on urination, and may be associated with symptoms such as urgency, frequency, and terminal dribbling.
- Acute retention: causes dull lower abdominal pain with inability to pass urine.
- Dysuria: pain on passing urine. Can be a non-specific sign. May be described as burning or stinging, and can be associated with many other symptoms, for example pain in the abdomen in cases of appendicitis, or signs of sepsis in patients with pyelonephritis. May radiate to the lower back in upper urinary tract pathology.
- Torsion of testis: acute onset severe pain in the testicle or lower abdomen. Can be associated with nausea and vomiting or swelling of the scrotum. May happen spontaneously or following a history of minor trauma to the testicles.
- Flank pain: pain in the flank may be linked to many disease processes; urological, orthopaedic, and general surgical. Pain associated with fever/rigors, urinary frequency, and a positive urine dip can be indicative of pyelonephritis, abscesses or pyonephrosis. Pain associated with gross haematuria and a palpable mass in the abdomen can be indicative of malignant disease, although this is now an uncommon finding due to improvements in imaging and diagnosis at an early stage.
- Non-specific pelvic pain: may be due to several surgical and medical diagnoses. Careful history taking and examination may point towards a diagnosis, however this may be difficult as pelvic pain is a very non-specific symptom. Important factors to consider when taking the history are whether the pain is linked to any potentially life threatening pathology, such as ectopic pregnancy or appendicitis. The possibility of sexually transmitted infection and pelvic inflammatory disease should be considered in all patients, and history taking should cover this area.
- Pain associated with urogenital tumours: many urogenital cancers are not painful when they first arise. The pain that patients experience may be due to the local effects of the tumour (for example renal tumours may cause pain by stretching the renal capsule), metastasis (especially common in late stage prostate

cancer, where up to 90% of patients will experience pain from bony metastasis), or due to the treatment given, whether it be medical or surgical.

- Pain associated with urogenital trauma: loin, abdominal, pelvic or external genital depending on the site of injury. It can also be related to associate non-urological lesions.
- Paraphimosis and priapism: localised penile severe pain with a considerable psychological impact.
- Fournier's gangrene: remember that pain may improve whilst the gangrene advances leading to an almost certain death.

Once a thorough history has been taken to assess the cause of pain a treatment strategy can be formulated. The first objective is to establish the severity of the pain in order to assess the effectiveness of treatment and the amount of analgesia which is likely to be required.

Analogue pain scales.

The analogue pain scale is a method of quantifying pain in order to assess treatment efficacy (Fig. 10.1). This can be simply achieved by asking the patient to place their pain on a scale of 1 to 10, with 1 being virtually no pain and 10 being the most pain that can be experienced. To make this clearer for patients a visual analogue scale can be used. This can either feature numbers to quantify the pain, or it can be used as a line of a standard length with no numbers, which the patient can mark to monitor treatment progress. If the use of a numerical scale is a problem, for example patients at extremes of age and those with special educational needs who struggle with numeracy, the scale can be altered to use facial expressions to convey the severity of pain. Examples of these scales can be seen below.

The WHO analgesic ladder was initially developed to guide the treatment of pain in the care of cancer patients. Once the severity of pain has been assessed the patient can be started on the stage of the ladder which corresponds to their pain severity. This ensures that an appropriate amount of analgesia is administered. If the pain severity changes the patient is moved up or down the ladder according to their needs.

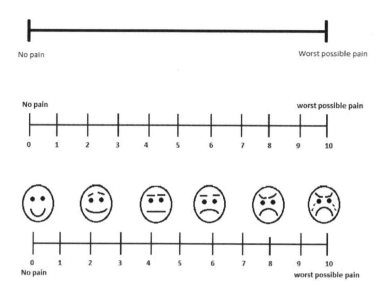

Fig. 10.1. Examples of visual analogue scales for pain.

3. Methods of Analgesia.

The choice of analgesic takes into account many factors. The severity of the patient's pain should be considered, in addition to the site and cause of the pain as some analgesics are particularly effective at treating pain caused by, for example, smooth muscle spasm or neurological involvement. The patient's age, weight and comorbid conditions should be considered, as pre-existing respiratory, cardiac, renal and liver disease may have implications on the choice and dosing of drugs. Potential interactions with any medication the patient is already taking should be considered too, with particular reference to psychiatric medication as many drugs interact with commonly used analgesics. As all drugs have potential side effects, the analgesic management plan should aim to treat the pain effectively using the lowest possible doses of appropriate medication. Analgesics can be broadly divided into opioids, non-opioids, and adjuvants to pain management and the management of severe pain may require a combination of all three options to optimise analgesia.

Non-Opioids.

This category of pain relief includes simple analgesics, such as paracetamol and NSAIDs. They are useful in the treatment of mild to moderate pain, and may also reduce the requirement for opiates in severe pain.

Paracetamol: the most commonly prescribed analgesic. It can be given intravenously, orally and rectally. Unclear mechanism of action, thought to work on COX-3 receptors in a similar way to NSAIDs. Effective for the treatment of mild to moderate pain, also has an antipyretic effect. Caution in patients who are malnourished, have liver problems, and people with alcohol dependence. Usual dose: 1g every 4-6 hours. Paracetamol can cause hypotension when rapidly administered intravenously, it should be given as a slow infusion over 15-30 minutes to counteract this.

NSAIDs: includes drugs such as Diclofenac, Naproxen and Ibuprofen. These drugs reduce pain caused by inflammation by inhibiting COX-1 and 2 enzymes. They also have antipyretic properties. Possible side effects include gastric irritation and ulceration, which can lead to major GI bleeding, bronchospasm and renal failure. Most drugs can be given orally; some NSAIDs can also be given intramuscularly, intravenously and rectally. Particularly useful in the management of renal colic. Caution must be exercised when using NSAIDs in patients at risk of, or with known, renal failure. This is due to the effect of the drugs on the synthesis of prostaglandins. In healthy individuals, prostaglandins cause vasodilation of the afferent arterioles of the glomeruli. In patients with renal failure, in order to maintain the glomerular filtration rate (GFR), there is an increased level of angiotensin II which constricts both the afferent and efferent arterioles. This deleterious effect if offset by the action of prostaglandins, which dilate the afferent arteriole, maintaining GFR. As NSAIDS reduce the production of prostaglandins, the result is unopposed arteriolar constriction in the afferent arteriole, which leads to a reduction in GRF. This effect is exacerbated by dehydration, and by concomitant use of ACE inhibitors and diuretics. Doses: Ketoprofen: 1 to 2 mg per kg every 6 to 8 hours. Maximum 300 mg per day. Ibuprofen: 400-600 mg every 8 to 12 hours, recommended daily dose: 1200 mg, maximum dose 2400 mg per day. Ketorolac: high analgesic potency, 10 to 30 mg TDS, maximum dose 90 mg daily.

Opioids.

Used in the treatment of moderate to severe pain. Strong opioids in particular are very effective analgesics, but have a wide side effect profile. Some examples include Morphine, Tramadol, Fentanyl, and Oxycodone. All opioids cause respiratory depression and reduce gut motility to varying degrees, leading to significant constipation. They can also cause nausea and vomiting, euphoria, CNS depression, bradycardia and hypotension. Opioids have also been shown to cause contraction of the urethro-vesical sphincter and relaxation of the detrusor muscle, which can result in urinary retention. Because of the multiple undesirable side effects opioids should be used in the lowest doses possible to provide effective analgesia, and should normally be augmented with non-opioid analgesics as discussed above, to reduce the opioid requirement as much as possible. The principle of dosing of opioids is careful titration, with close monitoring for both response to treatment and the occurrence of side effects. All opioids in common use are excreted by the kidney, and therefore caution should be taken when treating patients with renal failure, and expert advice sought when appropriate.

Codeine: weak opioid, given orally as a single drug, also available in combination with paracetamol for convenience. Pro-drug metabolised to morphine in unpredictable way due to genetic differences in enzyme expression. Pronounced antitussive effect. 30-50 mg TDS or QDS.

Morphine: most common strong opioid. Can be given orally, IV, IM, and rectally. 0,1/mg/kg. Can cause significant nausea and vomiting, especially at high doses. Use anti-emetic.

Fentanyl: strong opioid with a potency 100 times that of morphine. Used in the management of severe pain- can be given IV, orally in the form of lozenges and lollipops and transdermal. Can also be given as epidural analgesia, in combination with local anaesthetic. Metabolites are not active, therefore may be an alternative to morphine for patients with renal failure. 1-2 mcg/kg/hr by continuous IV infusion.

Tramadol: weak mu agonist, analgesic effect by inhibition of serotonin reuptake at the spinal level. Fewer side effects and is generally well tolerated. Can cause dizziness and vomiting. Dose 1 to 2 mg/kg every 6 or 8 hours. Maximum dose 400 mg per day.

Adjuvants to analgesia.

When pain control remains an issue despite adequate oral analgesia there are several options available to augment the delivery of pain relief. The first step in the control of difficult to manage pain should be to involve the acute pain team. Once it has been established that additional pain relief is required beyond that suggested by the WHO analgesic ladder (Fig. 10.2), the two most common options are epidural analgesia and patient controlled analgesia (PCA).

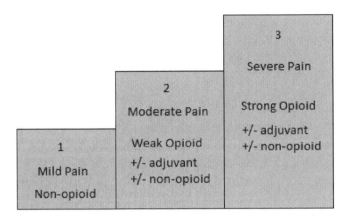

Fig. 10.2. The WHO pain ladder, showing treatment progression.

<u>Patient controlled analgesia:</u> this is a system whereby the patient is connected to an intravenous supply of opiate (usually Fentanyl or Morphine). The patient has a switch which is connected to the pump and can deliver themselves small bolus doses of the analgesic when required. There are several advantages of this system. For example it gives the control over analgesia to the patient, reduces the nursing burden for difficult to manage pain, and allows the pain team to assess the patient's opioid requirement. The pump also must have a built in "lock out" system, which limits the number of doses a patient can give themselves in a given time period (usually one dose every five minutes), limiting the potential for accidental overdose. The major drawbacks of this system are that some patients may find the system difficult to use, either due to a physical inability to use the button (e.g. patients with rheumatoid hands), or because they do not understand or remember how to use the button (the elderly, those with post op confusion, and people with severe learning difficulties). It may be difficult to set a programme for patients with opioid tolerance leading to potential under- or over-estimation of analgesic requirement. The system also requires a dedicated IV cannula, and fluids should be run at the same time as the PCA to prevent pooling of the drug in the cannula and to ensure efficient delivery. Other considerations include the need for monitoring for signs of respiratory depression, Naloxone should be prescribed to treat this, and supplemental oxygen provided at all times to prevent hypoxia should it occur. Patients should not be on any additional sedatives or

opioid drugs while they are connected to a PCA, and should be prescribed non-opioid analgesics like Paracetamol and NSAIDs for their opioid sparing actions. The patient should be reviewed regularly by the pain team to ensure that they are using the PCA appropriately and that the programme is effective and adequate for their needs.

Epidural analgesia: this is a form of analgesia that requires the insertion of a soft plastic catheter into the epidural space. This procedure must be undertaken in strictly aseptic conditions by a trained operator. The catheter can remain in situ for up to five days, and can be used to give either bolus doses or continuous infusions of local anaesthetic, which can be combined with an opioid. This system can also be operated by a patient controlled system, where by a background infusion rate is augmented by patient controlled bolus dose. A correctly sited epidural offers excellent analgesia, and may be particularly suitable for urological patients who have had open surgery. They have also been shown to reduce the incidence of post-operative respiratory tract infection and possibly MI, probably due to the reduced physiological stress and improved mobility offered by good pain relief. There are, however several potential drawbacks to this route of analgesia. The catheter itself may be difficult to insert, and once sited does not always offer a predictable level of analgesia. Patients may complain of a patchy distribution of block, sometimes dermatomes, or even a whole side of the body may remain unaffected by the block. There is a risk of permanent nerve damage, infection and bleeding during insertion of the catheter. Once the epidural has been successfully sited, the most common problem is hypotension, which can be profound. This is due to peripheral vasodilatation due to loss of sympathetic tone, and should initially be treated with IV fluids. Hypotension may occasionally require treatment with vasopressors and invasive monitoring in HDU. Patients with an epidural in situ are often unable to urinate normally; therefore most patients should be catheterised to prevent urinary retention. There is also a small risk of respiratory depression and excessive sedation when an opioid is used. Because of the many potential risks to the patient, frequent observations should be taken by a member of the nursing staff. These should take into account the patients vital signs, in addition to the level of block, pain scores and an assessment for nausea and vomiting. This level of observation means that most wards have a cap on the number of epidurals they can accept, and patients are frequently nursed in high observation areas.

Acute pain team: a major management point in the care of patients with either epidural or IV PCA is the involvement of the acute pain team. This is a team made up of anaesthetists and nurses with specialist knowledge of the management of pain. They often can offer advice and support regarding hard to manage pain, and are able to initiate PCA and epidural analgesia. Most hospitals also offer an acute pain review service, where all patients with an epidural or IV PCA are reviewed daily to ensure that their analgesia is adequate and appropriate.

Summary.

Pain management in urological surgery is a potentially complicated area. The varied nature of pain in these patients, along with their co-morbid problems can make managing pain challenging. A systematic approach to assessment of pain, coupled with a stepwise approach to treatment with input as appropriate from the acute pain team should ensure a good starting point when managing these patients. This will facilitate treatment, with reduced complication rates and an overall more positive hospital experience for the patient.

Additional reading:

1. Systematic review of the relative efficacy of non-steroidal anti-inflammatory drugs and opioids in the treatment of acute renal colic. Holdgate A, Pollock T. BMJ. 2004 Jun 12; 328(7453): 1401.
2. Prostate cancer pain management: EAU guidelines on pain management. Bader P, Echtle D, Fonteyne V, Livadas K, De Meerleer G, Paez Borda A, Papaioannou EG, Vranken JH. World J Urol. 2012 Oct; 30(5): 677-86.
3. Pain and its treatment in urology. Tenti G, Hauri D. Urol Int. 2004; 73(2): 97-109.
4. Heid F, Jage J. The treatment of pain in urology. BJU Int. 2002 Sep; 90(5): 481-8.
5. Comprehensive treatment of chronic pain by medical, interventional, and integrative approaches: the American academy of pain medicine. Deer TR, Leong MS, Buvanendran A, Gordin V, Kim PS, Panchal SJ, et al. New York: Springer; 2013. p1104.

Afterword.

This book came out of need. We needed to have a simple guide to manage patients with Acute Urology problems in secondary and tertiary care. We did not want that information to be diluted into physiopathology. We wanted straight answers at our fingertips.

I believe the hard work of our team did something meaningful towards that goal.

Mr J Clavijo.

Index.

[1] With permission from EAU.
[2] With permission from Dr R Molina Escudero.

[3] Modified from: www.glowm.com.
[4] Courtesy of Dr A Fahmy.
[5] With permission from EAU.
[6] With permission from EAU.
[7] Courtesy of Dr M S Runyon.
[8] With permission from EAU.
[9] With permission from EAU.
[10] With permission from EAU.
[11] With permission from EAU.
[12] Modified from: primary-surgery.org.
[13] Modified from: uro-plovdiv.com.
[14] Modified from: Keio University Hospital.
[15] Modified from: Dr I Gill.
[16] Modified from: Ternopil University.
[17] Courtesy of LearningRadiology.com.
[18] Courtesy of Dr Z Ansari.
[19] Courtesy of Dr P Jha.

49771617R00137

Made in the USA
Middletown, DE
21 June 2019